THE NEW ANXIETY

THE NEW ANXIETY

Emotional Problems during the Pandemic of Covid-19

César M. Garcés Carranza, Ph.D

Ordering Information:

For orders and inquiries, please contact:
1-888-404-1388
www.goldtouchpress.com
book.orders@goldtouchpress.com

Printed in the United States of America

Contents

The Social Worker as Facilitator with Relatives of Persons Infected with Covid-19

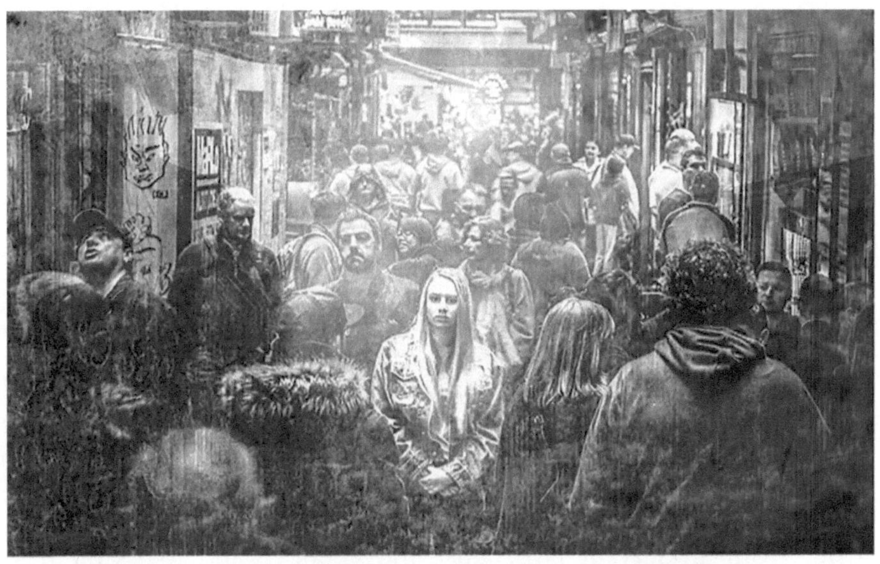

The dreams of a person who has been traumatized by the Covid-19 more than they have been in years. A girl cannot concentrate on school or at home, scared that her grandparents are going to get infected with Covid 19. A person who has obsessively stopped washing his hands has backed down in the middle of a public message service walk ordering him to do the same thing. The coronavirus can be serious and also fatal, especially for the elderly, minors, and people with other medical conditions such as (asthma, diabetes, heart problems), may be more vulnerable to seriously getting sick and dying.

People may experience:

1. Cough
2. Fever
3. Tiredness
4. Difficulty breathing (in severe cases).

For millions of people with post-traumatic disorders, obsessive-compulsive disorders, and other forms of anxiety are debilitating, the Covid-19 is causing a growing threat to mental health. All this started when it appeared on the news that "a new thing is in the environment, a new virus." People heard the alarm and immediately began to see things in the environment and saw them as a threat. The new Covid-19 and the fear of the respiratory problems it causes, have alarmed people of all kinds of social lives from all over the world. Most people are worried and afraid about this epidemic that has already become a pandemic.

For most people suffering from anxiety disorders, the effects of Covid-19 can exacerbate this debilitating condition. This can result in a trigger for many people, especially those who suffer from obsessive-compulsive disorder or worry about getting sick and stressed of having to worry about something new can exacerbate symptoms of obsessive-compulsive disorder and post-traumatic disorder or trigger more frequent panic attacks in people of higher risk. When people suffer from anxiety, it is because they believe and focus on lies, distortions and exaggerations in their imagination.

We see the image of Covid-19 everywhere, and this fuels anxiety in people. We see the news in big letters "THE FIRST PERSON TO DIE ON LONG ISLAND!" This sounds scary, anyone suffering from anxiety disorder, including anxiety disorder cares about this virus. Since the outbreak of Covid-19 came out, 100% of this author's patients have expressed fear, anxiety, even panic of contracting the coronavirus and for this reason they are afraid to leave their homes.

The fear that Covid-19 can cause in people who have anxiety tendencies may develop this debilitating disorder. Chances are that, for many people with conditions of anxiety, they are going to start to feel worse, we are not going to end up with short-term cases of virus, with this we are also going to end up with many cases of unrest or anxiety.

Some tips for people diagnosed with anxiety disorder and for those who are watching news on TV or Facebook:

1. Keep up the routine as much as possible.
2. Avoid the groups.
3. Sleep, this is good for the immune system.
4. Eat healthy food, avoid junk food.
5. Do not drink too much alcohol or coffee.
6. Exercise, it will calm you down and increase the immune function.
7. Read news from trusted newscasts.
8. You do not get absorbed with the news
9. Rests, practice table games, watch comedy TV preferably.
10. Listen to your favorite music, have fun while able to do it.

Emotional reactions of family members:

When a person becomes ill with Covid-19, and dies, emotional reactions are crushing, especially for the immediate family (parents, siblings, grandparents, children, wife, girlfriend, brothers, grandchildren, nephews, uncles, and cousins). Because much energy is focused on the sick, those people may seem invisible, as if they did not matter. While all the attention is focused on the sick, relatives do not realize how difficult the situation is for them as well. Also, keep in mind that the attention of a loved one should not be lost in the process. Keep in mind that the person caring for the patient also has emotional reactions such as:

1. Anxiety.
2. Fear.
3. Unger.
4. Frustration.
5. Fault.
6. Anguish.

Relatives of the sick person need to:

1. Being treated with respect.
2. Participating in the medical care of the loved one.
3. Be honestly informed about the condition of the loved one.
4. Be free from physical and emotional pains.

Testimony of a woman about her elderly mother:

"My mother passed away last May 2018, almost two years before the pandemic of Covid-19. I had been her sole caregiver until I had to place her in a nursing home in 2017. Her care had become too much for me to handle alone and her health situation needed intensive nursing care that I could not provide. But I was with her every day. We laughed and talked, and I held her hand when she was anxious and afraid. I was with her when her health crashed, and she passed away. I new her passing was inevitable, but still it hit me hard. I was not ready to let her go. I felt guilty that her last year was in a nursing home facility, and not in her beloved home of 66 years, the home she built with my father after their wedding. That last day, Could I have done more? Did she hear me say I love you? Did I say enough? Should I have fought and told the doctors to do everything to resuscitate her even though they said they could not? By the

beginning of 2020, I was in a deep depression. To go anywhere, to do anything was hard, Although I knew I should. I forced my self to visit my kids and granddaughters I tried to be happy. I knew I was floundering that I should not just sit at home although, that was really all I wanted to do. I was still grieving but thought I should be better.

Then the pandemic of Covid-19 came, and we went into lockdown in March 2020. Most people hated it. For me it was an instant relieve. I did not have to pretend anymore that I was afraid and force myself to go out, which some days was a real battle. It had been exhausting. I had to stay at home. The lockdown gave me permission to stay home. No longer having that battle everyday telling my self I should be doing something was a relief. I also realized early in the lockdown that although my mother was gone, I did not have to worry about her in a nursing home with no visitors. I did not have to worry if she would contract the coronavirus. And not having those worries helped me free myself of guilt, I had carried for so long and although I still missed her greatly, I could finally let her go.

My experience in no way disregards the pain others have gone trough during this terrible time. I realize it has been hard for others to grieve their loved ones during such a time. But everyone grieves in their own way. For me, the isolation of the lockdown helped me to focus on positive memories and not of guilt that was weighing me down for so long. It was a time of healing that I so desperately needed.

It has been a year of lockdown. But most places are opening now. People are getting vaccinated and getting together again. Shopping, eating out and visiting family and friends. I had time to heal from a devastating loss. But being home was a safe place; safe to grieve and safe from the coronavirus. Once before I was unable to go out due to depression. Now I find myself afraid to go out because of a virus that could cause me or my family members to get sick or maybe die.

Family members are often asked to participate in life-or-death decisions, which can worsen the crisis between them. Every day we see in the news that people are dying from Covid 19 and it is necessary to maintain close communication with relatives. Obstacles must be overcome by providing effective interventions, especially with those who do not understand or speak English. Obstacles to good communication include different attitudes about medical care and misunderstandings that can interfere with communication.

To make an intervention plan and an adequate evaluation in these kinds of interventions, it is essential to help family members overcome stress and emotional crisis, as it could have positive results. Clinical social workers use in the content of crisis intervention, the ability to make a difference. Clinical social workers, based on the crisis intervention model, can assist relatives of coronavirus-affected patients by reducing trauma. The approach of clinical social workers is about what is happening in the present and not in relation to the past.

During these times of crisis, clinical social workers must be part of the interdisciplinary effort for crisis intervention. Clinical social workers can collaborate with the professional staff of the hospital. Crisis intervention is important for clinical social workers, especially in trauma situations such as what is currently happening with the pandemic of Covid-19. Providing adequate interventions to people in crisis situations and emotional stress is part of the daily practice of clinical social workers. Unfortunately, the intervention cannot be offered in person as in other circumstances where there is no risk of infection. Therefore, interventions can only be by video conference or by telehealth. As mental health professional, this situation could be frustrating and stressful mostly due to the inability to intervene properly since personal intervention is not the same as by phone or video.

Trauma and emotional disorders are the cause of different emotional effects on people. While death and danger are for many people, the most extreme situations are trauma. People feel similar emotional discomfort when faced with the challenges of everyday life, especially if they face something difficult for the first time and so the challenge seems to threaten certain areas of emotional weakness, which occurs in different ways, such as the case of Covid-19. A person's desperation and anguish may not be the cause of any threat to another person. This model reminds this author that other people's perception is different from ours, whether we are the ones who are dismayed, or the ones who are helping someone else to deal with the problem.

Social workers provide emotional support to patients' relatives. Clinical social workers have an opportunity for crisis intervention with patients' relatives. Clinical social workers are constantly challenged to demonstrate their clinical skills and in the same way, they also could influence other health professionals and the public. All of us, at a given moment in our existence, will have to face tragedies, epidemics, disasters, and crisis situations that can then become emotional traumas, difficult to overcome, for example, the death of a loved one (parents, children, brothers, grandparents). The practice of clinical social work involves a process that determines professional intervention, regarding what needs to be done, how to do it and in what order, to ensure that people can overcome the obstacles that afflict them.

In short, the intervention of social workers in crisis situations is important for the following reasons:

1. Identifies and control crisis situations.
2. Provides crisis interventions.
3. Promotes interventions to relieve specific symptoms and reduces the risk of emotional stress.
4. Assess the environmental reaction and connect the victim (patient), family and caregivers (doctors, nurses), with available community resources.
5. Identifies psychosocial interventions.
6. Evaluates and manages psychosocial aspects of pain/penalty.
7. Assess the effectiveness of crisis intervention.

What needs do relatives of patients infected with Covid 19 have?

Based on this author's professional experiences, (Bronx Lebanon Hospital Center, Queen County Neuropsychiatric Institute, Flushing Hospital Outpatient Mental Health Clinic, and Community Counseling), in crisis situations patients' relatives have several needs. These are grouped into areas that are universally experienced by most people:

1. Receive security; reflecting the need to maintain hope and talk about the recovery of the sick. Meeting this need can promote trust, security, and freedom of doubt.
2. Staying close to the family; reflecting the desire to unite and maintain the positive relationship of the family. Satisfying this need can help the family calm their fear.
3. Receive information reflecting the understanding of the condition of the sick person. Meeting this need lays the groundwork for family members to make decisions and help the sick person.
4. Be comfortable; reflecting the need to reduce emotional stress. When comfortable, energy is conserved, fear and stress are reduced.
5. Receive emotional support, reflecting the need for professional intervention or assistance. Meeting this need helps relieve stress, anxiety, improve the resources available to the family and maintain strength to support the sick person.

Communication with patients' relatives is an important component of clinical social work. Relatives are given the opportunity to ask questions, to express their concerns, their fears, their feelings, and emotions, without fear of being judged. When a person is sick and has no emotional capacity to make medical decisions and is likely not to recover, the role of the clinical social worker is to locate his or her relatives or acquaintances and inform them about the patient's admission to the hospital and, at the same time, to find out if the patient has ever spoke to them or about his/her medical wishes in case he/she could not do so.

The following individuals may consent to medical treatment if the patient does not have the emotional capacity to do so:

1. Wife (legally married).
2. Fathers.
3. Adult children.
4. Brothers.
5. Adults who know the patient.

The clinical social worker recognizes and respects the dignity of people. The clinical social worker also, works with multiple systems and is attentive to individual differences, resolving conflicts that are consistent with the values, principles of ethics and norms of the social work profession. Meeting with family members is important to achieve an honest discussion about the patient's goals and desires regarding the necessary medical care. With the emotional support of the clinical social worker can achieve control, predetermination, connection, concentration to be able to make decisions that mean for the family.

As a facilitator, the clinical social worker must be engaged in the interest of the patient and his family, have communication skills, be an expert in conducting meetings with families, understand the group work process, have preparation in family dynamics and finally can focus on emotional questions and answers within important activities. The time and duration of the meeting with family members vary due to the number of members present, the complexity of the situation, the time required for family members to express their emotions, their fears, and to gather enough additional information from medical staff.

Although many of the resources and communication guides are available, one of the most practical ways to facilitate communication about their emotional content was described by Kira, P and Kira, J. (2004), Garcés, C. (2018):

1. Being fair.
2. Maintaining the course of communication.
3. Give time.
4. Show that people are important.
5. Covering adequate information.

Currently, there are not formulas that meet all the emotional needs of relatives of patients. The clinical social worker tries to gather the necessary information and recommendations from the medical staff, along with the emotional needs of family members and their process of understanding, to increase the sense of control, connection and meaning. Within this context, the patient receives the medical care he/she requires, while family members will be willing to learn defense mechanisms to control their fear, grief, for the possible loss of their loved one. The clinical social worker plays an important emotional support and collaborative role in maintaining constant communication with family members and medical staff (facilitator).

Proper clinical social work intervention with patients and family members who speak only Spanish, or another language requires a firm understanding of two complex languages, as well as the skills of being able to communicate efficiently in any language and in different situations. Patients and family members are unsent, in-experience, and may suffer outcomes that could be dramatic when confronted with inherited stress in the context of Covid-19 disease or any other disease.

Clinical social workers who do not speak the same language as the patient or their families (Spanish in this case), may face significant challenges during the interview and evaluation. These challenges include:

1. Inadequate communication.
2. Inadequate provision of services.
3. Inadequate definition of problems and needs.
4. Lack of adequate understanding of the individual's functioning and family dynamics.

The assessment of different situations and needs of patients and their families can result in serious problems due to lack of understanding of the ethnic-cultural and socioeconomic content. Interview and evaluation difficulties can also occur when the clinical social worker does not have the proper academic training to deal with people from different ethnic and cultural groups.

Situations that trigger crisis situations in clinical social work:

1. Frustration of not being able to intervene in crisis situations.
2. Disappointment of the profession for not providing the necessary elements to generate change.
3. Disappointment in the patient for not following the advice.
4. The clinical social worker blames himself/herself for not being able to help.
5. Loss of control.

Meetings with the relatives of patients admitted to the hospital prove to be an effective way for them to discuss emotional aspects and difficult decision-making. Clearly, the most intense of these is the decision to discontinue the medical treatment of a loved one. Exploring the patient's values and desires with the family in a private place, where there is enough time for them to express their emotions and discuss difficult topics, can create an environment of trust. These meetings are important because shared information about the patient can be heard by all members of the family present. This is also the right time for them to express their emotions (sadness, anger, fear, joy), feelings (scare, pain)and show emotional support "by touching" verbal expressions of affection.

For some family members, this may be the first time they have been allowed to think and talk about the reality of the patient's condition. The main objective of the meeting with the patient's family is to ensure that the patient's wishes are respected, that his relatives are aware of these wishes, that they recognize that everything that must be done for their recovery has to be done and that the medical staff will do everything possible to save the patient and his/her recovery. The clinical social worker must clearly explain the reason and desires (wishes)at the beginning of the meeting. For example, the social worker can say to the family: "Here you are to talk about the values and desires (wishes) at of your loved one, to discuss and explain his/her medical condition, what is happening with the patient now, the implications of his/her condition, especially the prognosis of his/her recovery, and to enforce together the patient's decision regarding the steps to follow based on the recommendation of medical personnel."

Medical and psychosocial problems domain are connected to the health system. The psychosocial field of clinical social work is the basis for creating a new partnership with patients, families and medical staff. The challenge for clinical social workers is to be able to demonstrate the relevance of their professional, emotional, intellectual ability and clinical skills to understand and address the emotional needs of patients and their families. Being able to control the emotional and spiritual reactions of patients and their families is the basis for effective clinical intervention.

Meeting with patients' relatives is important for being an excellent vehicle for creating an honest communication environment, focused on mobilizing the resources that are available to help the patient and their families towards a mutual action plan.

Conclusion:

From the author's academic training as a clinical social worker, he has learned directly and indirectly many messages that make him an excellent professional and fortunately today has a different understanding that allows him to live and practice this profession better. Perhaps despite the possible dissatisfaction of many professionals, difficulties persist in clinical social workers to make a difference between:

1. Giving the best we have and do the best we can.
2. Rest is necessary to regain energy, reduce emotional stress and regain professional efficiency.

All these advantages acquired by the intervention of clinical social workers in crisis situations have the possibility of promoting mental health to patients, their families, and medical staff. People outside the social work profession have the possibility of not being familiar or informed about the skills of clinical social workers. Lack of knowledge and understanding of what clinical social workers do can create conflicts in collaboration with other health professionals in providing services for their patients. The efficient intervention of clinical social workers in crisis situations depends, in part on other professionals and how the public perceives clinical social workers.

The challenge for social workers is to be able to demonstrate the relevance of their professional ability and clinical skills to improve the emotional condition of relatives of patients affected by Covid-19. Clinical social workers must contribute to research initiatives, not only to demonstrate the efficiency of the profession and intervention, but also to promote recognition among colleagues in other professionals about the importance of identifying and communicating the emotional needs of family members. Clinical social workers must understand that they play an important role during these times of global health crisis created by Covid-19.

Before we are clinical social workers, we are sensitive people, vulnerable to pain, fear, sadness, rejection, and many other feelings.

Emotional Problems
The Challenge for Social Workers:

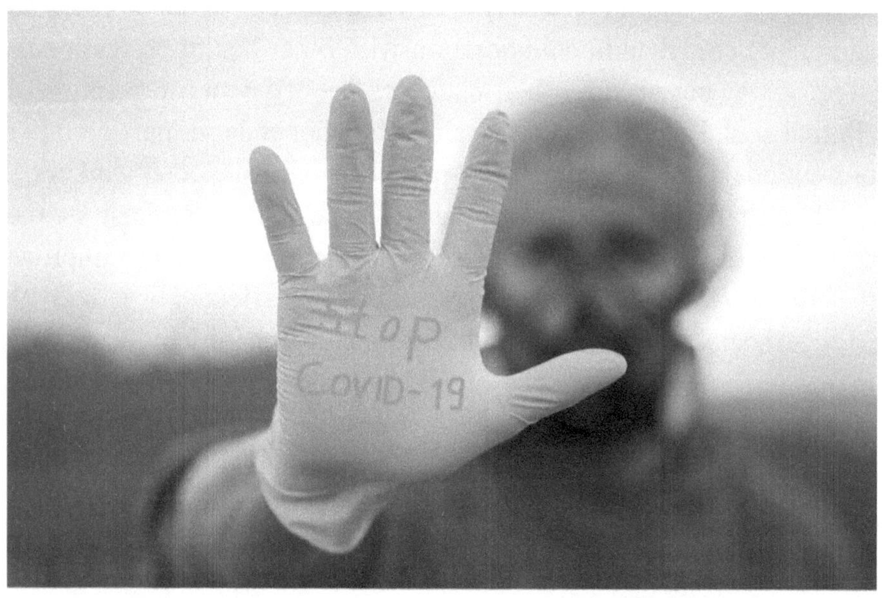

   While access to technological access is an option, clinical social workers report loss of economic income due to reduced attendance of billable sessions. Many people are losing their jobs in numbers never seen before, which impacts access to health insurance, co-pay funds for the cost of sessions, and the limited way to pay by phone or internet plans to participate in telehealth. When social workers can connect with their clients/patients, they often find that they must expand the time of their sessions to serve their clients/patients so that they learn how to navigate the telehealth system, the time spent that they will not be able to bill and what could cause them to have a few hours left to be able to care for additional clients/patients. In addition to the risk of income reduction, these low-paid social workers often struggle with their expenses that are associated with the telehealth system, such as the high expenses related to the data plan used for internet access and the need to acquire or update technology or equipment, such as computer and other equipment to work remotely.

For social workers, being able to provide telehealth services from home is a privilege. New programs show that some clients/patients can talk to their social workers/psychotherapists in their cars and in private. To protect the privacy of clients/patients, some social workers are offering telehealth services in their bathrooms, sitting in the back yard of their homes, or in their cars. For those social workers with children and other dependents, finding someone to help them with their children is not an easy task, nor is it an option, due to financial, health or logistical reasons. As a result, social workers are constantly redefining what multiple tasks mean so that they offer effective clinical services and juggle interruptions and decrease background sound.

This is the reality that many clinical social workers in mental health are facing. As a profession, we must begin to recognize and value the physical and emotional well-being of our workforce. Social stating protocols have been established, hand washing and to continue to wear protective equipment (mask, gloves). Some mental health-focused companies have made their products available and free to mental health professionals and hospitals are prioritizing initiatives that support the recovery and provision of mental health by clinical social workers (Lai J, Ma S, Wang Y, and colleagues, 2020). In this profession already challenged due to high numbers of rotation and emotional exhaustion, additional stressors can cause more clinical social workers to leave the profession, thus destabilizing the physical and mental health system during the time of the impacts related to the Covid 19 pandemic and could increase needs to the top and resources at the lowest.

Clinical social workers are superheroes at the center of the pandemic. As clinical social workers we must be aware that, during our dedication and courage, we also face difficult realities that are exacerbated by the disparities of our own lives. It is our duty to support each other during this difficult time and ensure that our mental health system survives these challenges intact and that it can be recovered.

What will be the new wave of Covid-19?

Probably after having been locked up and isolated for a long time affect people's mental health. Social isolation and confinement can lead to a list of mental health problems, so people face a way of living with restrictions due to the pandemic of Covid-19. Social isolation, as well as uncertainty about how long the pandemic will last, could contribute to increased anxiety and depression.

Humans are social beings, and need interaction with others. Side effects of the pandemic response will have an impact on people's mental health. Anxiety is high, so is depression. We all know that economic problems are challenges for individuals and families and confinement and social isolation can contribute to several mental health problems such as depression, anxiety and can also cause high risk of illicit drug and alcohol use, domestic violence, child abuse, as well as post-traumatic disorders. People suffering from mental health disorders are at risk of decompensation caused by the impact of Covid-19 (anxiety-depression). Stress, related to joblessness and childcare, can put many people at risk. Education about the risk of mental health problems is important to avoid emotional problems.

It is in the author's opinion that post-traumatic disorders will be the new wave of this pandemic and he also believes how important it is to erase the stigma about emotional problems because it can happen to anyone, especially in these pandemic times. It is important for our mental health that we focus on the present and relate to friends and family through social media. In the meantime, social gatherings must be avoided.

The Impact of Covid 19 on Social Workers' Mental Health:

According to the Kaiser Foundation (2020), in a mental health system that often has many challenges and few resources, the Covid 19 pandemic has been the cause for increased mental health needs around the world. The World Health Organization (WHO) pandemic impact models project an uptick in these needs in both acute and long-term results of this crisis (WHO, 2020). To respond quickly and continue vital services in the continuing changes in the changing reality of spreading isolation measures, governments and health insurance companies have quickly aligned to adjust telehealth policy. These changes have been adopted relatively effectively in systems that are financed, which already have a telehealth infrastructure, such as some hospitals. Although, in many systems, disparities integrated into the mental health workforce have a profound impact on their ability to implement telehealth so that they work around the clock to focus on increasing the needs of people during the Covid 19 pandemic.

Tips for parents of children and teenagers during the Pandemic of Covid-19

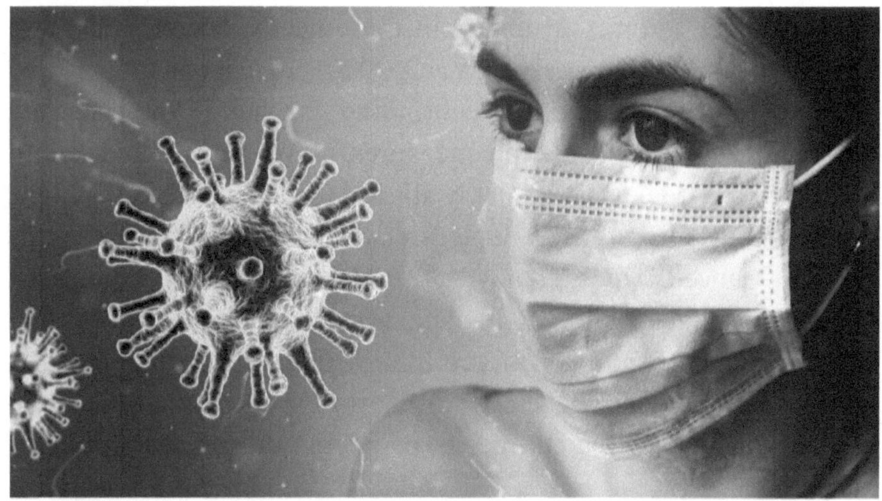

Covid-19 is a major epidemic. Hopefully, few children will get sick. Most sick children will have moderate cases. However, children are being affected by quarantine and anxiety and stress from their parents and other adults. Adults may think that children do not realize all the changes and stress caused by Covid-19 coronavirus, but they are sensitive to what is going on. Here are some of the ways kids react to stress and some of the thing's parents can do to help them.

Common ways children react to trauma:

1. They cry frequently
2. Difficulty standing still, calm

3. Problems with too much sleep and little sleep
4. Nightmares (can repeat what they have heard, pay special attention to their doll and hide them).
5. Some children may behave aggressive and angry
6. Others may want to use the battle instead of the cup to drink their milk.
7. Some may behave like babies, and forget how to use the toilet
8. Others will want the bottle instead of the glass of milk
9. Others may want to eat soft food.
10. Talk like babies.

Children are overly sensitive to their parents' stress experience. This affects their ability to act in their usual way and affects their emotions. Children often cannot talk about their fears or their anguish. Babysitters can protect them from adult stress, but adults should realize when children are upset.

What can parents do to help their children during the epidemic of Covid-19?

Routine is important for children. Disasters create isolation and other traumatic situations disrupt daily routines. By creating new routines or re-establishing usual routines, Parents can help children feel safe and secure. Keeping the feeding time scheduled, sleeping, organizing time to play together, reading them a book, or singing songs together, all of this can help.

1. The support of parents or caregivers is particularly important during times of stress and during the time after the disaster has passed. Parents may not be physically and emotionally available because they themselves are stressed too. Therefore, it is the importance of making time to reassure children and spend more time with them.

By explaining why things are different, young children may understand why things have changed (as they cannot leave the house to play) but talking to them will help them feel protected by their parents.

1. Children should be helped in a way that is age appropriate.
2. Keep explanations simple
    Even if children are not directly exposed to trauma, they can realize and stress and worry other siblings and adults in the house. Even if children are not directly exposed to trauma, They can get stressed and worry other older siblings and adults in the house.
3. If the children have been sent to be with other family members elsewhere, in another home, it is important to speak to them using electronic means of communication as often as possible during the day and at bedtime. If the children are in the house parents must try to make plans for them to communicate with other children (friends), either by phone or videos. So, the measures of social stating wear out, much has been written about how children are dealing with this pandemic. Little has been written about teenagers, who are missing great opportunities (the end of classes, undergraduate graduations, promotion of year or school, playing sports, parties, visiting with friends). As well as deprived of basically doing what they say is "full time": separating their parents, exploring new places and starting to realize who they are.
4. A recent survey, conducted by Harris Poll on behalf of the 4-H National Council (2020), 7 out of 10 teenagers said they were somehow having problems with their mental health. More than half said they had had anxiety, 45% said they had been over-stressed and 43% said they had been depressed. By some context, 12% of American teens meet the depression criterion and about 30% gather the anxiety disorder criterion by the time they turn 18.

5. Based on the results of the survey that according to Jennifer Sir Angelo, president, and chief executive of 4, H, "the Covi-19 has had an adverse impact on adolescent mental health (2020)." For example, 61% of the adolescents interviewed said that the Covid-19 pandemic has increased their sense of loneliness." These results indicate increased stress and concern in mental health, like the experiences of older adults. A recent John Hopkins study conducted in April (2020), comparing how older adults felt during 2018 on the same date, showed a triple percentage increase in older adults suffering from symptoms of psychological distress.

6. An important result of this study is that teens reported that during the pandemic they spend at least nine hours on their device screens, an increase of at least three hours a day. The study could not establish the cause and effect, but according to the experts it is certainly reasonable to expect that all the time on the devices could increase the feelings of teenagers. One of the respondents responded when they announced the results of the *study:*

7. *"The coronavirus has been quite overwhelming and being in social media has sometimes been a lot for me."*

8. To some extent, teens have been required to be on their devices most of the time to be able to get classes remotely. This learning model may very well continue next school year. It is the opinion of this author, the important thing that is that the parents of the students spend as much time as possible with their children when they are not using their devices. Although many students may be making use of their devices most of the school day and during recess, it is also important that parents spend time with them. These interactions are important for strengthening connection, creating routine, and providing personal interaction that could not happen otherwise.

9. It is also important that parents are in direct contact with their children and not be intimidated to ask them questions when they want to know something about them. Ask them if they are having trouble with something or someone. Perhaps talking to them about their own emotions or problems could help to try to connect and start a conversation without threats. Teenagers usually like this kind of communication, according to the study of (The Harris Poll, 2020). At the same time, 80% of respondents said it might be uncomfortable to ask for help.

10. Despite the general picture described by this study about how teenagers deal with Covid-19, there are reasons to be optimistic. Generally, children have the emotional ability to recover early, and this study found something similar: Nearly 70% of the teens in the survey responded that they were able to recover soon. This is a positive sign for teens to feel confident and able to face obstacles. There are ways parents can implement to boost their children's ability to overcome themselves, such as helping them focus on what they have control over and creating a space between them so their children can talk freely about their emotions.

It is not easy to anticipate a scenario where teenagers can find, but we can equip them with certain skills and skills so they can navigate this complicated and overwhelming world. More importantly, teenagers know it is okay and there is nothing wrong with asking for help.

What can parents do to help their teenage children continue to browse this challenging situation that doe not seem to end soon?

1. Resisting the need to save your children
2. Let them discover their own ways to deal with and solve their problems
3. Focus on supporting them in their projects

4. Helping them talk about their emotions
5. Highlight what they can control
6. Be a model of flexibility
7. Let them know it is a long way to go

In addition to claiming lives and our livelihoods, the Covi-19 crisis has disrupted almost every aspect of our daily lives. Not only that, but the pandemic has also torn apart all the communal meetings that would otherwise have helped us deal with the grief, uncertainty and fear it has brought us. The pandemic affects us all equally and everywhere in the world. The pandemic is insidious, silent, and invisible. We do not know how much to finish, or how much the human and economic cost will be.

It is exceedingly difficult to deal with our fears and our emotions when the world we met is no longer and will not be the same.

Anxiety, Depression in Times of Covid-19

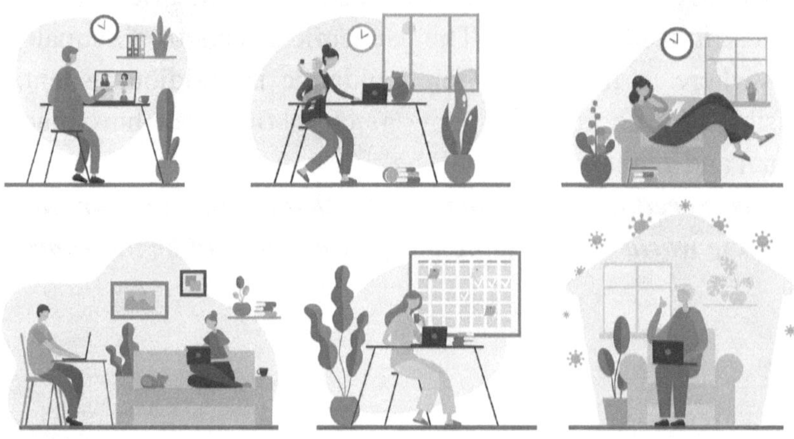

The pandemic of Covid-19, coronavirus has caused emotional problems of anxiety and depression in the American and Latin American communities. Not only has the number of cases increased, but the waiting time to make an appointment with a clinical social worker (psychotherapist) or a psychiatrist has also increased. For many these symptoms are derived from the loss of loved ones, loss of employment, and financial problems and social isolation. According to a report from the Center for Disease Control (CDC, 2020), anxiety and depression symptoms have increased considerably in June 2020, compared with the same period in 2019.

In the community mental health centers where this author practices psychotherapy, have seen an increase of patients who have been referred by their primary care physicians, usually reporting problems with sleep or fatigue, anxiety, and depression. Also, reporting symptoms such as headaches, back and muscle pains, sadness and worried about their families. Based on his professional experience with the Latino communities, to talk about mental health is often misunderstood with "being crazy."

Anxiety is ubiquitous; anxiety disorders are not. Anxiety is an unpleasant and unjustified sense of apprehension often accompanied by physiological symptoms, while anxiety disorder connotes significant distress and dysfunction due to the anxiety (Tom, D., 1995). An anxiety disorder may be characterized by only anxiety, or it may display another symptom such as phobia or an obsession and present anxiety when the primary symptom is resisted (Tom, D., 1995). Fear is also universal and can produce the symptom picture of acute anxiety states, yet in contrast to anxiety, the cause is obvious and understandable (Tom, D., 1995).

Types of Anxiety (DSM-5, 2013):

1. Chronic, Mild Anxiety:

Tension, irritability, apprehension, and mild distractibility are common (particularly in medical and psychiatric patients), often related to environmental factors, and treated with supportive and reality-oriented psychotherapy.

2. Chronic, Moderately Severe Anxiety:

Is more severe, chronic anxiety (longer than six months, usually years but waxing and waning) and including symptoms such as autonomic responses (palpitations, diarrhea, cold clammy extremities, sweating, urinary frequency), insomnia, poor concentration, fatigue, sighing, trembling, hypervigilance, and/or marked apprehension. It tends to run in families, has a moderate genetic component, and is associated with simple and social phobias and with major depression.

3. **Acute Anxiety-Panic Attacks:**

Has dramatic acute symptoms (peak within 10 minutes) lasting minutes to hours, is self-limited, and occurs in patients with or without chronic anxiety. Symptoms are perceived by the patient as medical and are characteristic of strong autonomic discharge-heart pounding, chest pains, trembling, choking, abdominal pain, sweating, dizziness, as well as disorganization, confusion, dread, and often a sense of impending doom or terror. Attacks may come "out of the blue" or may be initiated by crowds, stressful situations, or anticipation (anticipatory anxiety).

4. **Anxiety with Specific Fears:**

Phobias are fears that are persistent and intense, are out of proportion to the stimulus, make little sense even to the sufferer, lead to avoidance of the feared object or situation, and when sufficiently distressful or disabling are termed a PHOBIC DISORDER. Common, mild, frequently transient fears (of the dark, heights, snakes) receive no diagnosis. Phobias may wax and wane over months or years and may disappear spontaneously, but serios cases may continue for decades and gradually take the form of a depressive disorder. The fear may generalize during their developing stages, of, fear of a store generalizes to the street front the store and then to the entire shopping area.

5. **Agoraphobia Without History of Panic Disorder:**

Multiple phobias with chronic anxiety: specifically fear of open and /or closed spaces, unfamiliar places, being alone, and more generally, of a loss of a sense of security. Many other fears and hypochondriacal concerns may be present, as well as multiple other symptoms including fainting, obsessional thoughts, depersonalization (feel unreal, detached), and derealization (feel surroundings are unreal). Depression is common. This is the most disabling phobic disorder.

6. Social Phobia:

Fear of scrutiny from others during public speaking, using public lavatories, blushing, eating in public, etc. Typically begins during adolescence. Some patients are troubled by specific and limited social activities while others suffer from generalized social exposure. Marked general anxiety is common in severe cases: Patient controls by avoidance-can be socially crippling.

7. Posttraumatic Stress Disorder:

If a patient suffers a severe loss or stress (rape, serious car accident, harm to a child or spouse, natural disaster, combat, prison camp, etc.), he/she may develop the clinical syndrome of Post-Traumatic Stress Disorder. A mixture of the following symptoms is present initially:

a. Market anxiety,
b. personality change with irritability and poor concentration,
c. an exaggerated startle response,
d. insomnia and nightmares,
e. intrusive thoughts of the event,
f. reliving the feelings experienced at the time,
g. avoidance of anything associated with the trauma,
h. emotional blunting which can impair interpersonal relationships and day-to-day functioning,

Later, depression, emotional numbing, and preoccupation with the trauma may predominate. The more severe the stress, the more likely PTSD is:

1. To develop trauma,
2. to be long lasting,

It may resolve after months (last 1-3 months=acute) or, untreated, last for decades (more than 3 months-chronic).

8. Acute Stress Disorder:

Is an expected reaction of anyone experiencing an adequately severe trauma, yet the individual requires different amounts and types of stress to develop it. PTSD symptoms predominate:

a. nightmares,
b. reexperiencing the event,
c. avoiding stimuli that remind one of the traumas,
d. irritability,
e. hypervigilance,
f. poor concentration, and
g. marked startle response.

9. Anxiety Disorder Due to a General Medical Condition:

Medical conditions (most commonly cardiac disorders) can produce anxiety states, although often they generate no sense of apprehension or foreboding. Other medical conditions can produce an anxiety syndrome:

a. intracranial tumors,
b. menstrual irregularities,
c. hypothyroidism,
d. hyper and hypoparathyroidism,
e. post conscious syndrome,
f. psychomotor epilepsy,
g. cushing's disease.

10. Substance-Induce Anxiety Disorder:

Almost any drug of abuse can produce an anxiety syndrome on intoxication, while anxiety symptoms commonly predominate upon withdrawal from alcohol, hypnotic-sedatives, and cocaine. Similarly, several medications can produce anxiety with use: eg,

a. antihypertensives and cardiac drugs,
b. thyroid,
c. sympathomimetics and bronchodilators,
d. anticholinergics,
e. antiparkinsonian meds,
f. lithium and,
g. antipsychotics medication.

Once the cause is identified and corrected, the anxiety usually promptly disappears.

11. Anxiety with Obsessions and Compulssions-Obssessive Compulsive disorder:

Obsessions are repetitive ideas, images, and impulses that intrude upon a patient who feels powerless to stop them. They are unwanted, distressful, occasionally frightening, or violent (eg, the impulse to leap before a car; the thought that he/she may attack his/her spouse), and often impair functioning. The patient can ruminate endlessly ("did I lock the door?"); most people develop rituals or compulsions (counting, touching, cleaning). The cause of OCD is unknown, but CNS serotonin neurons are implicated in some cases.

During the pandemic, things do not seem to be all clear and it is not easy for many parents when the schools were opened. Before the pandemic, the students had the support of their teachers and guidance counselors. All of this has changed and is complicated. The academic needs are enormous and complex and now there is an academic gap between students of higher and lower resources. Many students of low socioeconomic backgrounds do not have access to the internet or means of transportation to go to school or to go to the library as compared with those students from higher economic background.

For many parents and families of different socioeconomic levels, the academic learning from their homes is presenting countless challenges. From the ability to provide adequate space, quietness and silence so their children can study, to the lack of access to the internet. Lack of supervision from those parents who have to work outside of their homes, and the worried of not having enough knowledge to be able to help their children in the different academic levels that they attend.

For many children in public schools and of lower economic resources, the tutoring curriculum and additional cost that are seen in many communities of higher learning is not an option and this causes stress and worrisome for many parents. By not being able to offer additional tutorial or online education to their children, parents wonder if their children are really learning.

All these problems mentioned are real. Without counting the external challenges to education that many families have, such as the fear of eviction or losing their homes, insecurity of adequate feeding, the need to take care to their adult family members with chronic medical conditions. Also, lack of adequate medical insurance and the stress of having to work outside of their homes, perhaps in centers of employment where they can be exposed to the coronavirus is a threat to their health even to lose their employment.

It is now when clinical social workers should identify the different ways in what they can help and support people and families in need. The United States and the world are suffering emotional reactions that are frequently distressing due to the fear of the Covid-19, and in many cases, the fear of getting infected with this virus.

The outbreak of the coronavirus has caused more than 850,000 deaths and more than 86,000 million of confirmed infections since last February 2020. According to a report from John Hopkins University (09-2020), The United States totals more than 6 million cases, and about 198,000 deaths. This crisis has left many people without employment to millions of people, hit the economy and forced many businesses to close.

How to Take care of our Mental Health:

1. Focusing on what we have control.
2. Practice hygiene.
3. Have a routine to go to bed and to wake up.
4. Program time to do something and enjoy it.
5. Reminisce past pastimes.
6. Have a support system (friends/family).

Cultural Sensitivity in Clinical Social Work

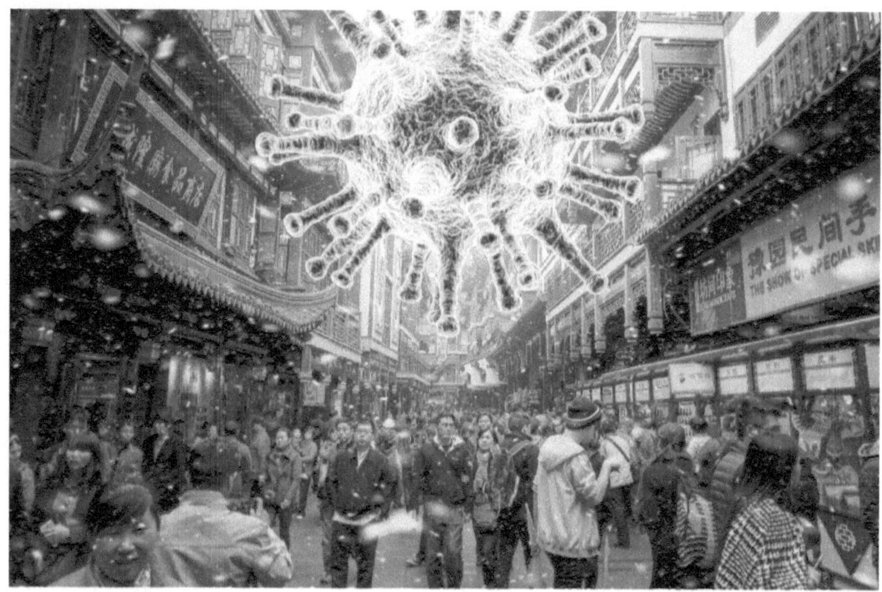

Cultural sensitivity in social work is knowing that there are differences between cultures, but without putting a value on differences (better, or worse, right, or wrong). It is easy for conflicts to occur at this point, especially if a custom or belief goes against the idea of multiculturalism.

The author seeks to describe the current context of his practice and that of other clinical social workers who work with clients/patients from a racial, ethnic, and multicultural background. There is an agreement in the literature that the ability of service providers to work with people from different cultures is important to clients/patients in minority ethnic groups. Clinical social workers play an important role because they are the ones who shape the cultural sensitivity of any prevention program in their professional life. Thus, the beliefs of social workers, values, world vision and ways of knowing are essential components in efforts to provide services that are authentic and culturally sensitive.

In addition to educational preparation in cultural competence (CSWE, 2015) and ethical requirements (NASW, 2017), a look at literature on minority clients/patients suggests that there are gaps in translation into practice. Individuals from racial and minority groups are less likely to receive high-quality mental health services (McGuire, T.G., and Miranda, J., 2008). Lack of minority representation among health professionals' results in low use of mental health services.

Few efforts have been made to develop knowledge related to the provision of mental health services. So far there is no empirical evidence related to cultural competence of mental health providers and the satisfaction and experiences of recipients of minority ethnic groups. Clinical social workers should understand that they play an important role in identifying and treating psychosocial problems.

I. Culture:

Is the set of material and spiritual goods of a social group transmitted from generation to generation to guide individual and collective practices. It includes language, processes, ways of life, customs, traditions, habits, values, patterns, tools, and knowledge (Imaginary, A., 2000). Culture influences all spheres of human life. Imaginary, A. (2000), defines health, illness and seeking relief from the distress caused by the disease. With increased mobilization of people across borders between countries and geographies, multicultural trends are emerging in many countries around the world. This is reflected in the cultural diversity that is presented to clinical social workers in their daily practice. With these presentations' patients bring their world opinions, expectations, standards, taboos, to the clinical transaction. Cross-cultural transactions occur when two or more of the participants are culturally different.

While it is impossible to converse with people from different cultures, clinical social workers should be sensitive to the role that culture plays in their practice without stereotyping patients. Culture has an influence on seeking help and this can be partial in the evaluation process and intervention model. Cultural exchange between client/patient, place of practice of the clinical social worker can create challenges in obtaining personal history and other factors such as age, ethnicity, gender, religion, sexual orientation, and acculturation.

II. Multicultural Social Work:

The concept of multicultural social work practice is extensive and includes different groups, such as women, men, ethnic and racial groups, people with physical disabilities, religion, minorities, sexual orientation, and others (Sue, D. W., Rasheed, M. N., and Rasheed, J. N., 2015). The practice of clinical social work with people from diverse cultures is influenced by different epistemologies that guide the way culture is conceptualized (Williams, C.C., 2006). From the critical perspective, culture is seen as a tool of power from one group to another (Williams, C.C., 2006). This definition of culture has been widely accepted in some parts of the world such as Latin America, which has been more critical of the oppression of power structures (Freire, P., 1970). In the United States, social work literature tends to describe culture predominantly in terms of values, beliefs, customs, and acculturation, often focusing on the context of clients, particularly economic disparities. From this perspective, culture tends to essentialize and pathologize and be used as a tool to hide structural barriers and limit the opportunities of life (Viruell-Fuentes, E.A., Miranda, P. Y., and Abdulrahim, S., 2012).

As socially respected professionals, clinical social workers have a responsibility to understand that they bring a system of cultural values to their place of practice. Their actions will have effects and impacts on the community and the people to whom they provide their professional services. A critical analysis of the systems of cultural values that clinical social workers carry within the space of encounter with clients/patients and how they reflect institutional values and structural systems, and ideologies, could ensure the provision of services to clients/patients who are culturally diverse.

Multiculturally competent clinical social work practice is important to ensure the effectiveness of access to treatment for this population. The importance of multicultural competence is reiterated in the (NASW, 1996) Code of Ethics. Cultural competence focuses on the need for sensitivity to cultural factors that may influence clients/patients (Colón, E., 1996). Being variably sensitive and multicultural can be conceptualized as sustaining a cultural lens of human behavior and making concessions for possible multicultural influence. However, to avoid stereotype, it is important that social workers recognize existence within the group's differences, as well as the influence of clients/patients' own personal and cultural values. Cultural competence is, at best, aspirational (Caldwell, L.D., Iwamoto, D.K., Tarver, D., and Herzberg, S., 2006), and requires the continuous development of cultural sensitivity and understanding, knowledge and skill of social workers.

As clinicians, social workers need to continue to work towards developing their knowledge base about changes in social dynamics. It is also important to recognize and understand that Latinos are not a homogeneous group. It can be argued that the same concept of the identity or affiliation of an ethnic group is problematic. Within the Spanish-speaking language, there are variations in diction, speech patterns, vocabulary, and vernacular use, each unique to its region of origin, the subtle tone in the voice can have different meanings within Latin cultures. For example, it is not out of the ordinary in Peruvian or Puerto Rican culture to speak out loud and this is often interpreted as shouting or fighting for those unfamiliar with these cultures. Understanding these differences is relevant to social workers working with this population. It is also important to understand that there are common points among many Latinos in the United States.

I. Concepts of Cultural Competence:

1. **Cultural Knowledge**: signifies that we know some cultural characteristics, history, values, beliefs, and behavior of another cultural or ethnic group.
2. **Cultural Awareness:** is the next stage of knowledge of other groups, being open to the idea of changing cultural attitudes.
3. **Cultural Sensitivity:** is to know that there are differences between cultures, but without putting a value on differences (better, worse, right, or wrong). It is easy for conflicts to occur at this point, especially if a custom or belief goes against the idea of multiculturalism. It is likely that, from time to time, an internal conflict (intrapersonal, interpersonal, and organizational) will arise in relation to this matter.
4. Conflict will not always be easy to manage, but it can be better done if everyone is aware of organizational goals. (The President's Initiative on Race., 1999).

II. Cultural Responsibility:

It is defined as the ability to meet the needs of a diverse group of people who are provided with equitable and quality health services. According to the National Quality Forum (NQF, 2009), cultural competence seeks to eliminate misunderstandings and improve patients' adherence to health treatment. The Office of Minority Health (2012) states that cultural competence is essential to avoid disparities in health services, because culture and language can affect someone's belief about: health, disease and cultures that lead to both. Being respectful of the responses of the individual and cultural needs of clients/patients, ensures more effective communication, in this way the needs of patients can be met. The Joint Commission (2012) recognizes the importance of patient-centered communication with its new standards, effective July 1, 2012, which mentions cultural competence. In addition, almost all hospitals and most physical and mental health providers are subject to federal civil rights laws such as Title VI of the Civil Rights Act of 1964 and the 1975 Against Age Discrimination Act. Organizations develop policies that guide employees to work within regulatory and legal guidelines. It is necessary to know and comply with these guidelines to avoid persecution. Cultural competence is not intimidating, as it recognizes and gives validity to people.

III. Development of Cultural Competence:

There is an important caveat to remember when developing cultural competence, which is not to make stereotypes. It is only a factor that forms the person, others include the environment, economic position, genetics, and psychological factors. Lack of knowledge about what is cultural competence does not excuse in that it requires being cared for by a same sex health care professional. The client/patient is examined by a health care professional who does not ask for his/her medical condition before the examination, this action may be inappropriate.

The health care professional's lack of understanding of the client's/patient's culture cannot deny the allegation cast by the health care professional. To better understand the definition of cultural competence, it is important to understand the meaning of the word *culture*. According to Chamberlain, S. P. (2005), culture represents "values, norms and traditions that affect the way a particular group perceives, thinks, interacts, behaves and makes judgments about the world where it lives." Nine-Court Carmen, J. (1984), defines culture to the set of human knowledge that includes behaviors, beliefs, attitudes, values, and experiences that are of immense value. This also includes different cultural structure. The benefit of cultural competence is that it eliminates racial and ethnic disparities by providing health services, including mental health.

IV. Integration of Cultural Competence in Psychotherapeutic Treatment:

Some examples that can be considered to help clients/patients and in the same way avoid misunderstandings and legal demands to health care providers (Nine-Court Carmen, J., 1984). In each case, the most important point is to provide acceptable options on the part of clients/patients:

1. Identify whether the client/patient has limited-based cultural situations about health care services by people of the opposite sex.
2. Determine if there are certain dresses or garments that clients/patients must wear.
3. Collaborate with clients/patients and family members to develop solutions and alternatives to orders that cannot be fulfilled.
4. Provide educational materials in the language of clients/patients.
5. Consider cultural influence on pain. In some cultures, the ability to withstand pain is of high value, so the client/patient does not speak when he or she feels pain. The clinician must take a closer look at the nonverbal signs of pain.
6. Verify written assessment tools for possible cultural biases that may affect the evaluation.

V. Obstacles in Cultural Competence:

Although language is important, this is not the only obstacle. Obstacles can be any aspect of health care that contributes to the misuse of health care. Obstacles can affect the quality of services offered and contribute to racial and ethnic disparities, which include, but are not limited to:

1. Lack of ethnic/cultural diversity in health facilities.
2. Health care centers are inadequately designed to meet the needs of the diverse population of patients being cared for
3. Communication problems between health care providers and patients from different ethnic, cultural, and religious groups.

Cultural competence is one of the ingredients to eliminate disparities in health services and it is for this reason that when clinical social workers and clients/patients talk about emotional problems without realizing the cultural differences that arise in their interaction, they intensify. To develop cultural competence, it is necessary to examine preferences and prejudices, looking for role models and sharing with people who have an interest in cultural competence.

The trainings provided in academic practice and internship typically do not have the formal standards and structures to ensure clinical competence in Spanish. Today, we witness the convergence of two inexorable forces initially separated: multiculturalism and evidence based on practice. These originated in different locations and were traditionally associated with disparate advocates (Journal of Clinical Psychology (2010). Interdisciplinary origins of psychotherapy include anthropological psychology, ethnopsychology, psychoanalytic anthropology (Comas-Diaz, L., 2011).

Demographic avalanche in the United States is incontrovertible. The most populous states will be transformed from mostly Caucasian to the majority of Latino and African Americans. Using U.S. Census data from 2005 to 2025, increases between Asians, African Americans, Native Americans/Eskimos, and Latinos are expected in all states except for Mississippi where the ratio remains the same (ww.census.gov/population/www/projections/natproj.html). By 2028, more than 50% of California residents will be Latino.

Cultural competence is an ethical mandate of social work practice and has the potential to increase the effectiveness of interventions by integrating the cultural qualities of clients (Jani, J.S., Ortiz, L., and Aranda, M., 2008). Competent social work incorporates diverse cultural bases, norms, and different ways of knowledge (kumpfer, Alvarado, Smith, and Bellamy, 2002; Moreno, and Bravo, 2002).

VI. Acculturation:

According to Torres, L., and Rollock, D. (2004), acculturation is one of the most studied adaptation variables and has been defined as changes in experiences by individuals having been in contact with other cultures. Acculturation is seen as a key to the variables that social workers should consider when working with people from different ethnic and cultural backgrounds. Acculturation is a process of dynamics and has been measured in different ways. Generally, acculturation has been measured in terms of behavior, cultural identity, knowledge, language, and values (Zea, M.C., Asner-Self, K.K., Burma, D., and Buki, L.P., 2003). These aspects are then critical components of understanding and addressing factors that cause intercultural conflict and distress related to the adaptation of the new culture

The people who adopt and integrate the values, beliefs and behaviors of both, host culture and ancestral culture are "bicultural." Despite the field of literature growth about acculturation between Latinos, the relationship between acculturation and distress remains complex (Torres, L., and Rollock, D., 2004). The study by Kaplan, M.S., and Marks, G. (1990), indicated that as levels of acculturation increase, distress also increases significantly in young adults, but decreases in older adults. These patterns were found consistent in both women and men and were independent of the effects of economic income and education. Simplistic understanding of the concept of "culture" for example, "high" vs. "Low" acculturation can lead to a weak explanation of health disparities and a deviant approach to structural constraints, such as racism and lack of access to resources (Abrador Lanza, A.F., Armbrister, A.N., and Flores, K. R., 2006). Cultural assimilation, also known as assimilation, is a process of consistent integration where members of an ethnocultural group (immigrants or minority groups) are absorbed into a generally long and established community. This presumes a loss of many characteristics of the absorbed group (Boyer, P. (2001).

VII. Health Care Disparities:

Non-Caucasian people are more likely not to seek mental health services until their symptoms are severe (Norris, F., and Alegría, M., 2005). People in minority groups are less likely to seek mental health services, but they tend to seek help from their primary care doctor or informal (botanical) support systems, family members, or friends. There are several reasons (Schwardzbaum, S.E., 2004). This, combined with the stigma usually associated with mental health concerns, decreases the likelihood of seeking adequate mental health services. Competent mental health services for Latinos and other minority groups consequently need to be easily accessible, have hours of care address communities, be perceived as credible, provide real referrals to other services, combine physical health services with mental health, client/patient feedback and have bilingual, culturally sensitive and compassionate professionals.

Doctors' offices, clinics, community mental health clinics, and hospitals see this diversity every day, and the need for culturally and linguistically competent health care services for diverse populations is attracting increased attention from health care providers and those who judge their quality and efficiency. While certain providers have delivered appropriate services to diverse multiethnic populations for many years, this has not been the case in many settings. As these settings begin to treat a more diverse clientele because of demographic changes, interest in designing culturally and linguistically appropriate services that lead to improved outcomes, efficiency, and satisfaction has increased. Unfortunately, many health care providers feel they do not have clear guidance on how to prepare for or respond to these situations. Up to this point, no comprehensive standards of cultural or linguistic competence in health and mental health service delivery have been developed by any national body.

VIII. Barriers in Health Care:

1. Language barriers are a major source of isolation and an obstacle to seeking health care and help for mental health problems.
2. Language barriers and lack of linguistic access services are significant barriers to care for people who do not speak the dominant language (English).
3. Non-English-speaking people may receive less optimal mental health care services than fluent English-speaking people.
4. Nonnative English-speaking people, even when speaking English, may have difficulty understanding frequently used medical terms.
5. Language difficulties are significant barriers to care for the Latino population.
6. Language barriers may result in inadequate explanation of medication side effects and decreased patient satisfaction with care.
7. Language barriers may contribute to disparities in treatment of patients with mental health problems.
8. The use of untrained translators can lead to distortions in the information obtained from the clinical interview.

XI. Skills Required:

The skills necessary for the culturally competent practice of social work are preached in the understanding of knowledge and values and the understanding of the applied values of the profession. Harper, K. V., and Lantz, J. (1994), developed an approach to cultural practice and social work sensitivity with all cultures seeking to transcend cultural variables. They identified eight factors that apply to practice with all cultures and ethnic groups:

1. Respect for the clients/patients world vision.
2. The importance of hope.
3. The assistant's conscience, such as affection, genuineness, and compassion.
4. The importance of trust.
5. Techniques designed to empower the client/patient, give them the opportunity to have control over their lives and their environment.
6. Initiation rites defined as rituals designed to deal with the stages of the transition of life.
7. Cleansing experiences (these are rituals designed to eliminate unwanted emotions).
8. Essential realization that means (helping the client/patient to seek purpose).

X. Professional Personal Use:

The practice of clinical social work with Latinos demands a careful personal evaluation and understanding of how clinical social workers see the world around them and how the dominant society affects their professional practice with Latinos. Therefore, social workers need to be aware of their own bias and how their world view affects their concept of clients/patients. For example, if a social worker's point of view is to value individualism, he/she should critically assess how to address a client/patient from a collectivist point of view (Furman, R., and colleagues., 2006).

The personal understanding of the clinical social worker is critical and involves the development of knowledge regarding cultural heritage and the effects of racial and cultural heritage, and history when working with clients/patients (Sue, D.V. and colleagues., 1992). It is important for clinical social workers to understand how class and classism can influence the course of therapy (Liu, W.M., and Ali, S. R., 2005). Therefore, being aware of the biases and perspectives as well as accepting that they are also partial and this can improve their effectiveness by working with clients/patients from different ethnic and racial groups that are different from theirs (Sue, D.V., and Sue, D., 1990).

Based on the author's professional experience, many Latinos patients' value intimate personal relationships. They also value the role of the clinical social worker and tend to adopt a "doctor-client/patient" tradition with the clinical social worker, especially at the beginning of the professional relationship. After graduating from Fordham University Graduate Program (MSW) and starting the practice of psychotherapy, this author was frequently referred to as "doctor." by many of his patients.

It is also important to understand why many Latinos would like to know about the personal/family life of the clinical social worker. As clinical social workers we must understand that this is not a matter of professional boundaries; the family is often critical of the view of the world surrounding Latinos and it is difficult to see a person outside their family context (Furman, R., and colleagues., 2009). Appropriate personal disclosures by the clinical social worker allows the patient to understand/the best as a person within the family context, thus cultivating a work alliance (Furman, R., and colleagues., 2009). During the first session, it is important for the clinical social worker to set boundaries and explain the process and treatment plan. Later, in the first session, the clinical social worker needs to foster the therapeutic alliance to convey affection and trust (Taylor, B.A., and colleagues., 2006).

Latinos have the same incidence of mental health problems when compared to the rest of the American population. Although it could be said that some experiences, ways of understanding and how they control them may be different. Without mental health, we cannot be healthy. Any part of the human body, including the brain, can get sick. We all go through different events or situations that can occasionally cause us ups and downs. Mental health problems go beyond the emotional reactions that pass through different situations. This has to do with some situations or conditions that could change our routine because they can get complicated and could create problems in relationships with some people, as well as in the place of employment and lose it. Without proper mental health treatment, problems can make a person's life worse and difficult (National Alliance on Mental Health, 2019).

Usually, Latinos do not talk about their mental health problems. There is not enough information on this subject, and we cannot know what they never taught us. Many Latinos do not seek treatment for their mental health, mainly because they do not recognize symptoms or because they do not know where to seek professional help or because of the stigma and fear of being called "crazy," as this could be a cause of shame. The cultural origin and characteristics of the individual play an important role in the etiology and psychological distress and mental health. It is known to many that minority ethnic groups are more likely to be exposed to the disproportionate single weight of a stressful experience. An example could be the experience of immigrants. Many immigrants (including the author), around the world having suffered varieties of traumatic experiences, including discrimination. Despite the immigration status, many immigrants suffer more acculturation problems as they try to adapt to the new cultural environment than those of the majority population (Williams, C.L., 1991).

Cultural assimilation is the process of gradually assimilating the characteristics of the new environment. This can also increase the risk of mental health-related problems so that immigrants are acculturated, possibly due to the regression of a prevalent narrative of incidences of mental health problems of the general population (World Culture Report, 2000). There is an increase in the research study indicating that U.S. born Latinos have greater evidence of a variety of physical and mental health problems than foreign Latinos (Rogers, L.-Sirin, and colleagues, 2014). In trying to unite the gap between cultural understanding and helping professionals systematically think about how to improve their treatment efforts, Hwang, Wei-Chin (2006) developed Adaptive Psychotherapy and Modification Framework (PAMA). The PAMA framework consists of three-staggered five broad domains, 25 corresponding adaptive and rational therapeutic principles. Adaptation domains include:

1. Dynamic problems and cultural complexities.
2. Guidance to clients about psychotherapy and increase the understanding of mental health.
3. Understanding cultural beliefs about mental health.
4. Understanding population-specific cultural problems.

This approach to presenting cultural adaptations to psychotherapy was developed to make the PAMA more accessible, easy to use and adaptable to be used with diverse populations. Although many effective treatments have been developed to treat mental health problems, little research has been conducted to determine their effectiveness with these groups from different cultural backgrounds. Recent reports suggest that people in minority groups are less likely to receive quality health services and that they show worse treatment outcomes, when compared to other groups. To improve care for those with diverse cultural backgrounds, Western psychotherapy could be culturally modified or adapted to be more effective in treating minority ethnic groups (Hwan, Wei-Chi, 2006).

Because clinical social workers in the mental health system need to be culturally competent, research and training to help them conceptualize and update these skills that are difficult to provide is necessary. Adaptation and treatment are especially important as the concept of therapy and the rationale behind therapeutic treatment could be culturally unknown to those clinical social workers with limited experience in mental health and cultures where mental health can be stigmatizing (Hwan, Wei- chin, 2006). Because many minority ethnic groups are culturally different from White Americans, the current health system may not be prepared to meet the needs of people's rapid diversity. This has become apparent as recent reports reaffirm that racial, ethnic and health disparities exist and that there are many disparities in the health system that can influence when people from different cultural backgrounds receive equitable health services (Smedly; 2003; USDHH, 2001). Concrete plans in presenting disparities in the health system at all levels need to be implemented. These plans need to be global and international in nature. Recently, the World Health Organization (WHO) reported says that five of the ten largest causes of disability around the world account for between 12-15% of the world's weight of disease (WHO, 2014).

In 2002, the American Psychological Association (APA) approved guidelines for multicultural education, training, research, practice, organizational change for Psychologists and clinical social workers (www.apa.org/practice/guidelines/multicultural.pdf). The guidelines are as follows:

1. It must be recognized that, as cultural beings, they can maintain attitudes and beliefs that can influence their perceptions and interactions with individuals who are ethnically and racially different.
2. The importance of multicultural sensitivity/responsibility, knowledge and understanding must be recognized about the ethnic and racial difference of individuals.
3. The importance of conducting ethnic and cultural research among people of different ethnic, racially minority, and linguistic stories must be recognized.
4. Appropriate clinical skills and applied psychological practices must be applied.
5. The process of organizational changes that supports culturally informed development and practice policies must be used.

12% of the population of the United States Speaks Spanish, making this the fifth longest Spanish-speaking country in the world (PASEO, 2019). This demographic struggle to obtain quality health services are due to the shortage of professionals who speak Spanish. Spanish speakers who are interviewed in English are often misdiagnosed, overmedicated, or pathologized. Many bilingual children are incorrectly placed in special education programs or do not have access to certain accommodations that are necessary learning with disabilities because of the lack of professionals who can do psycho educational and neurological examinations in Spanish (PASEO, 2019).

The multicultural cultural environment challenges clinical social workers to look like other people and to recognize that multicultural responsibility and adaptation lies not only in clients/patients, but that it involves everyone in the relationship (Marsiglia, F.F., and Kulis, S.S., 2009). To do this, clinical social workers need access to interventions and tools that have a culture-based approach. This approach begins by evaluating the existing opportunity for based and tailored interventions when needed, so they are more relevant to clients/ patients from various multicultural groups without compromising their effectiveness. This process of evaluation, refinement and adaptation of interventions will lead to a better equitable relationship of aid (Marsiglia, F., and Kulis, S. (2009).

According to Zayas, L.H., and colleagues. (1996), culturally sensitive intervention has been described as a continuation of the following dimensions:

1. Understanding of culture.
2. Acquisition and knowledge about cultural aspects (norms, customs, language).
3. Ability to distinguish between culture and pathology, and,
4. Ability to integrate the above dimensions into the intervention.

It is important to note that cultural sensitivity is a dynamic process that changes over time and in different contexts, in which the cultural hypothesis must be continuously evaluated against alternatives (Lopez, R., and colleagues., 1989). Over the years, several terms have been used to refer to the consideration of culture, including, "cultural sensibility," "culture centered," "culturally competent," "multicultural competition," or culturally receptive." All these terms, perhaps while varying in degree or intensity, have in common the consideration of culture and language and related problems in psychosocial intervention (Journal of Community Psychology, 2006). Over the past few decades, psychologists and other health professionals have called for the importance of considering culture and ethical and minority aspects in any psychosocial intervention (Bernal, G., and Sáez-Santiago, E. (2006). There is a need for the participation of minority ethnic groups in research, especially in the field of clinical social work.

Understanding culture's impact on mental health and its treatment is important, especially considering recent reports highlighting the realities of health care disparities and unequal treatment for minority groups. Recently, in the United States, The Surgeon General and the Institute of Medicine reported that social and ethnic health disparities exist, and in general ethnic minorities continue to be missing from the research from which evidence-based treatments (EBT) are drawn (Smedley, B.D.S., et al., 2003). In addition, there is a growing body of European and other international literature supporting these findings and suggesting that immigrants and ethnic minorities evidence a disproportionate burden of illness and unequal access to health care services (Department of Health, 2003). This accumulative body of evidence underscores the idea that extant health care systems may not be adequately prepared to meet the needs of minority and immigrant populations. The importance of incorporating issues of culture, race, and ethnicity into research, teaching, and clinical practice are really needed. This task has proven to be quite complicated given the limited resources that have been invested towards improving our understanding of cultural influences on mental health without guiding frameworks from which to work from, the larger audience of mental health professionals will continue to acknowledge that culture is important but struggle in articulating how culture makes a difference and be unprepared in addressing growing world-wide health disparities.

XI. Conclusion:

Whereas the emergence and advocacy for cultural competence within health grew from the ranks of community-based systems targeting ethnic-specific populations, it is especial that these systems do not become defunct as the health care system evolves. To achieve cultural competence within a system of care, collaboration across multiple systems is needed. While awareness of culture and the imperative of cultural competence has grown significantly over the past decade, there is still much to be done. Mission statements, goals and objectives need to be translated into action plans. Programs and services, and all aspects of the system of care including payers and regulatory authorities need to be evaluated and audited as to their level of cultural competence. Standards of culturally competent care need to be evaluated and audited as to their level of cultural competence. Standards of culturally competent care need to be mandated, developed, implemented, and monitored throughout the systems and across its multiple sectors. As we have shifted from cultural sensitivity to cultural competence, we now must shift to the development of standards and measurements of outcomes for cultural competence.

As the United States becomes a racially and ethnically diverse nation, clinical social workers need to respond to the diverse perspectives, values, and behaviors of the people they provide their professional services. Lack of knowledge and understanding of social and multicultural differences can result in negative consequences. Proper intervention requires for clinical social workers to have knowledge and understanding of the different sociocultural aspects of the people to whom they offer their professional services. This implies respect for both beliefs about psychosocial and emotional problems, as well as possible solution to their problems.

As clinical social workers, there is much to be done as mental health researchers, practitioners, and educators to improve multicultural sensitivity, and to incorporate cultural and linguistic competence, and to raise awareness about the impact of culture and language on health and mental health care delivery. As mental health providers, clinical social workers need to develop an understanding of how culture systematically affects the domains of mental health. Therefore, we must continue to promote strategies for creating environments in which people with emotional problems feel safe and able to control their lives again.

There is a need for the participation of minority ethnic groups in intervention and research, especially in the field of social work in mental health. University social work programs should create specific training programs that prepare students to provide effective interventions and practice in communities to solve complex psychosocial problems. They should also expand their institutional capacity to implement multidimensional service plans that respond to the multicultural needs and experiences of minority group students.

Understanding Mental Health

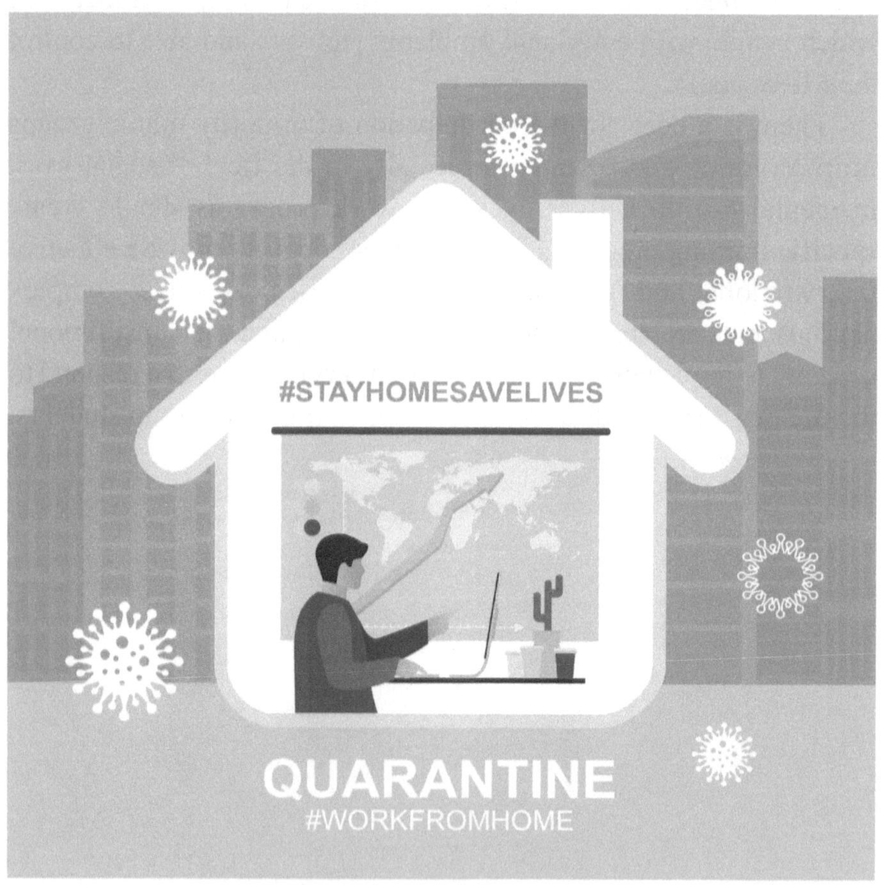

According to the World Health Organization (2020), mental health is a state of complete physical, mental, and social well-being and not just the absence of conditions or diseases.

Countries are introducing measures to restrict social movements as part of efforts to reduce the number of people infected with Covid-19. According the CDC (2021), 28,381.220 million cases of infection, and 500,000 people killed in the United States

More and more people are making changes to their daily routine. The new reality of working from home, unemployment, virtual education of elementary school, high school, and college. Lack of physical and social contact with friends, family and colleagues takes time to get used to this new way of living.

Long months of confinement can lead to psychological consequences in much of the population. Social isolation, confinement, and adaptation to new lifestyle. Changes like these, and controlling the fear of contracting the virus and concern about people close to us who are vulnerable, is challenging all of us without exception. This could also be difficult for people suffering from emotional disorders such as depression, anxiety, and compulsive obsessions.

Mental health is not only the absence of disease, but also the ability to develop respect for one's life. Mental health should be addressed not only from a physiological point of view, but also from a psychosocial (person-environment) point of view. What happens around the person that affects his/her emotional state? Therefore, mental health is important to overcome Covid-19.

Introversion/Social Extroversion:

Social anxiety is a disorder that can affect anyone, regardless of whether they are introverted or extroverted. However, the condition is more common among introverts. People who suffer from social anxiety fear being judged by their words or social behavior. This fear makes words or social behavior. This fear makes them doubt or be ashamed to speak in front of people, so that they do not say something socially wrong or behave in a way that can cause people to laugh at them or judge them. This fear can be mild and cause the person (introverted) to become nervous or paralyzed, preventing them from speaking.

Introverts enjoy spending time alone doing things like reading, drawing, painting, listening to music, etc. All these things allow the introvert to look inside and reflect on their own thoughts rather than focus on others. Introverts do not have to like being alone all the time, they do not mind leaving their house or with friends. However, they prefer to stay with a small group of friends, preferably with friends they already know.

Extroverts are people who like to talk to other people, go to parties and social gatherings, and enjoy other people's company, whether they are known or not. People extroverted during the Covid-19 pandemic can no longer socialize the way they used to. They are now limited to the use of technology (video conferences, cell phones, etc.). Instead, the introvert apparently does not feel much about change because he is used to being alone.

Tips for Maintaining Our Mental Health-

I. Stay Informed:

1. Listen to advice and recommendations from national and local authorities.
2. Follow news from trusted television channels, such as national radio and television, and keep up with World Health Organization (WHO) news.

II. Have Routine:

1. Get up and lie down at the same time every day.
2. Maintain personal hygiene.
3. Eat healthy foods.
4. Exercise regularly.
5. Make time to work and rest.
6. Make time to do rewarding things.

III. Reduce the number of news:

Try to reduce the amount of news you watch on TV and listen to news that can cause anxiety or stress. Search for the latest information at specific times of the day, once or twice a day if necessary.

I. Alcohol and illicit drug use:

Limit the use of alcohol (if you drink) or not drink it at all. Do not start drinking alcoholic beverages. Avoid the use of illicit drugs.

II. Social Contact is Important:

If your movements are limited, then you must try to maintain regular contacts with close people (family and friends) either by phone or online.

III. Time in front of the TV:

Be careful how much time you spend in front of the TV. You must take breaks from the activities in front of the TV/computer.

IV. Video games:

While videos can be a way to relax, these can be tempting to spend more time playing while in the house for long periods. Make sure you keep a balance with activities offline with daily routines.

V. Social Media:

Make use of social media to promote positive stories. Correct bad information when they are presented.

VI. Help others:

If possible, provide support to people in need in the local community, such as helping with food or food shopping.

VII. Support health workers:

You must have the opportunity to thank health workers and those who work by responding with Covid-19 cases.

VIII. Do not discriminate:

Fear is a normal reaction in uncertain situations. But sometimes fear is expressed in ways that can be harmful to other people.

Remember:

1. Be good, generous, do not discriminate against others for fear of catching the Covid-19.
2. Do not discriminate against people who have Covid-19.
3. Do not discriminate against health workers. They deserve to be respected and grateful.
4. Covid-19 has affected people in many countries without discriminating against specific groups.

IX. If you are a parent:

In times of stress, it is common for children to seek more attention from their parents.

What can be done?

1. Maintain family routines or create new ones, especially if they are going to be home.
2. Talk about Covid-19 with children honestly and they can understand, using age-appropriate language.

3. Help children with learning at home and make sure they have time to play (inside or outside the house).
4. Help children find positive ways to express their emotions, fears, and sadness. Sometimes when doing creative activities, such as drawings or playing, it can help children with this process.
5. Make sure children are away from TV screens every day and try to get them to do other creative activities together. Play, listen to music, draw, build something (models).
6. Prevent children from s passing more time than necessary by playing videos.

X. If you are an adult:

1. Maintain regular contact with family and parents, friends (by phone, email).
2. Maintain regular routines and schedules as much as possible, before meals, sleep, and activities you enjoy.
3. Do simple exercises while at home and in confinement to maintain body mobility.
4. Find out how to get help if necessary, how to call a taxi, or ask for food delivery or medical care. Make sure you have enough medications. Ask family, friends, or neighbors if necessary.

XI. If you have any medical or mental health conditions:

1. If you are on psychiatric treatment or medical conditions, be sure to take your medications and have enough medicine available. Keep in touch with your therapist, psychiatrist, or family doctor.
2. If you are being treated for drugs/alcohol, you are informed about Covid-19 that may cause increased fears, anxiety, and social isolation, which may cause the risk of relapse, drug/alcohol abuse, lack of follow-up treatment and regimen

ordered by doctors, especially if you are taking methadone and make sure you have enough medications.

3. If you are being treated for games continue your treatment.

XII. Meditation and Mindfulness:

Find a place where you can sit in silence and not be disturbed for a few moments (10 minutes). Start by drawing your attention to the present moment, focusing on your breathing. Pay attention to your breath when it enters and leaves your body. Before long, his mind will begin to wander, taking him out of the present. Take note of your thoughts and feelings as if you were an outside observer watching what is happening in your brain. Consider it and let yourself return to your breathing.

Social Isolation and its Effects on Sleep

According to studies by Elke Van Hoof (2020), social confinement is the greatest psychological experiment in history. It is estimated that, in March 2020, at least 2.6 billion people were placed under some form of quarantine. This represents one-third of the world's population. By mid-June 2020, Covid-19 disease had already recorded more than 9 million confirmed cases and killed at least 470,000 people. Some countries in Europe and Asia began to relax their confinement measures, but in Latin America many continue to have severe restrictions.

Studies on the pandemic of Covid-19, this is a global public health emergency with impacts on the mental health of the population. The pandemic is causing multiple psychosocial consequences (unemployment, economics) and psychological problems (anxiety, depression, post-traumatic stress disorder), as well as sleep disturbances.

According to the report by Altena, E., & colleagues (2020), the wakefulness cycle is contingent on multiple factors, mainly exposure to daylight and nighttime darkness. The latter increases levels of melatonin (a hormone whose function is to regulate the onset of sleep. Other factors influencing are meal schedules and daytime physical activity, the latter represented in both low activity levels and mandatory depression or confinement, such as high levels of activity due to stress, overwork or intense nighttime exercise negatively affect the sleep pattern (Altena, E., & colleagues, 2020).

Stress involves greater psychological and physiological activation in response to daily demands and it is known that the increase in hypothalamic-pituitary-adrenal axis (HHA) function is associated with short, fragmented sleep, with a possible reduction in sleep stage (Akerstedt, T. (2006).

Similarly, a short sleep causes increases in levels of stress-related markers, such as cortisol and, therefore, sleep disorders can create greater activation of the HHA axis, thus exacerbating a vicious circle between stress and insomnia (Akersestedt, T., 2006, Zhang, C., 2006). Sleep function is to regulate emotions, some alteration in the sleep pattern can have direct consequences on the emotional functioning of the next day, so that insomnia can increase anxiety levels, since people with sleep problems have a decrease in cognitive evaluation or with the cognitive approach of an emotional event to mitigate the impact (Kirwan, M., Pickett, S.M, Jarret, N.L. (2017).

Poor sleep quality can also increase negative emotions after disruptive life events and decreases the beneficial effects that are obtained from vital events with positive connotation (Kirwan, M., Pickett, S.M., Jarret, N.L. (2017). Insomnia is associated with suicidal ideas and attempts, this being a risk factor that can be modified (Kirwan, M., Pickett, S.M., Jarrett, N.L., 2017). Suicidal ideas are exacerbated by the conditions of social isolation and confinement. Insomnia is one of the most influential vaticinators in suicide attempts, like the existence of a specific plan to commit suicide (Escobar, F., Quijano, M., Calvo, J., 2017).

People who are exposed to stressful situations such as the Covid-19 pandemic can cause increased likelihood of anxiety, depression, as well as interruptions in the sleep pattern. Previous studies on social isolation and the psychological impact on sleep quality have highlighted in the following factors (Altena, E., & colleagues, 2020):

1. Decreased exposure to sunlight.
2. Dietary changes.
3. Ambient temperature by confinement.
4. Reduction of social interaction.
5. Work more hours under stressful circumstances.
6. Living with uncertainty and insecurity about mental health.

Every day, almost every media outlet has stories about the Covid-19 pandemic. Radio and television programs have uninterrupted coverage over the latest death figures and, depending on who you follow, social media platforms are full of scary statistics, practical advice, or black humor. This constant bombardment of information can cause anxiety, fear, depression, panic, with immediate effects on people's mental health.

Fear of contagion makes us more conformist and less receptive to eccentricity. When there is fear of a disease such as Covid-19, we become more vigilant and become judges of the behavior of others. Fear of the spread of a disease can cause prejudice and xenophobia to people we consider to be different from us. In addition to becoming stricter judges among people within our social group, the threat of disease can also make us more suspicious of strangers.

Some situations can be inducing significant stress, such as sharing a limited space where there are pre-existing family difficulties that can precipitate crises and for the elderly and those living alone. Confinement is likely to exacerbate loneliness and abandonment (Altena, E., & colleagues., 2020).

Those with stress-related sleep pattern interruptions are more likely to develop chronic insomnia (Akerstedt, T., 2006), and pre-existing insomnia is also a relevant risk factor for the development of post-traumatic stress disorder (PTSD) when people are exposed to stressors (Gerhman, P., & colleagues., 2013).

Recommendations for Maintaining the Wakefulness of Sleep Cycle:

Cognitive sleep therapy is appropriate for insomnia, classically aimed at treating chronic insomnia problems. Positive results have been seen to effectively treat acute insomnia, modifying stress-generated situations (Altena, E. & colleagues., 2020., Zhang, C., & colleagues., 2020), including a variety of psychotherapeutic components such as sleep hygiene education, relaxation psychotherapy, stimuli control, sleep restriction and cognitive re-evaluation (Altena, E., & colleagues., 2020).

Among the recommendations of sleep hygiene for confinement (Altena, E., & colleagues., 2020) are:

1. Ensure exposure to sunlight for at least thirty minutes during the day to improve melatonin production.
2. Do not drink caffeinated coffee or tea at night.
3. Reduce alcohol consumption.
4. Avoid exercise immediately before bedtime.
5. Ensure an optimal ambient temperature to fall asleep.

"If we do not respond quickly to any problems people may suffer, then we'll have a time bomb. (Elke Van Hoof, 2020)."

XIII. Conclusion:

For many, the Covid-19 pandemic, confinement, and social isolation have caused emotional disorders (anxiety, distress, depression, fear, panic attacks). Similarly, health workers in hospitals (emergency rooms, intensive care), doctors, nurses, paramedics, fire fighters, social workers, these are the first to provide emergency care to those infected with the virus. In the case of social workers, they provide emotional support, crisis interventions to the relatives of Covid-19 victims.

Cognitive behavioral psychotherapy for insomnia and other Covid-19-related emotional disorders is one of the interventions that can help people overcome dream problems, anxiety, depression, and panic attacks, which are exacerbated by stress related to confinement and social isolation.

Requirements to Succeed in Social Work

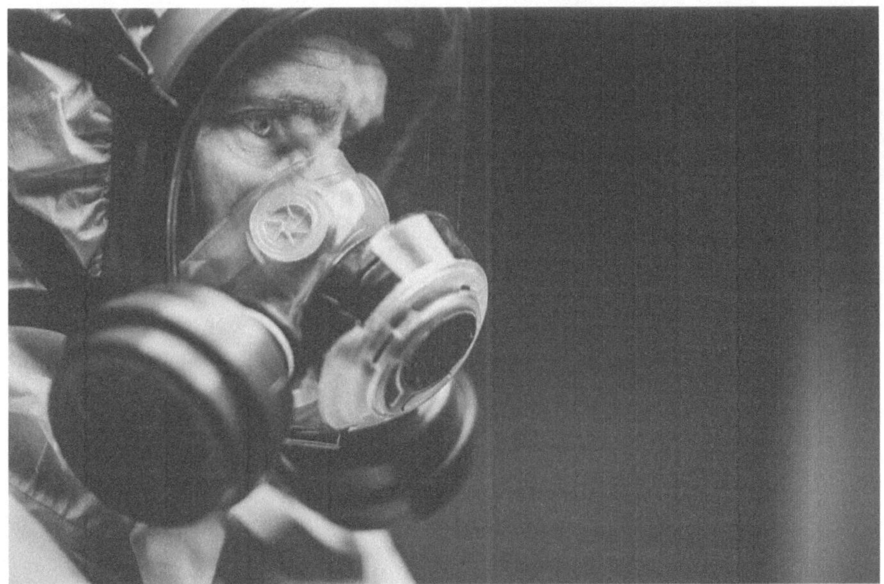

Social Work: is an academic discipline and profession whose interest is the well-being of individuals, families, groups, communities, and society, with the effort to meet basic needs and improve social functioning, personal determination, collective responsibility, and the total well-being of people.

Ten requirements for success in social work practice:

1. Empathy.
2. Communication.
3. Organization.

4. Critical thinking.
5. Actively listen.
6. Personal care.
7. Cultural competition.
8. Patience.
9. Professional dedication.
10. Advocate.

1. **Empathy:** Is the ability to identify with an understanding of the point of view of other people's experiences. The National Association of Social Workers (NASW, 2003) defines empathy "as the act of perceiving, understanding, experiences, and responding to another person's emotional state and ideas." Putting yourself in someone else's shoes and recognizing those world experiences, perceptions, and views and unique that allows clinical social workers to understand and build together a strong relationship with their patients. This is a vital skill that helps social workers determine the needs of clients/patients based on their unique experiences to provide efficient services. Barker, R.L. (2003).

2. **Communication:** (Verbal and nonverbal), it is a vital skill for clinical social workers. The ability to communicate clearly with a wide variety of people is essential. In addition to being cognizant to body language and other nonverbal signs, this means having to communicate appropriately and effectively with clients/patients regardless of their cultural history, age, sexual orientation, intellectual level, physical or emotional disability. Clinical social workers should also communicate with other providers, colleagues, and agencies and should clearly document and report information.

3. **Organization:** Clinical social workers have a busy schedule of responsibilities to others to serve and support multiple clients/patients, including documentation, bill reports, and collaboration. This requires that clinical social workers must

be organized and able to prioritize the needs of patients to handle cases. Disorganization and poor administration can cause the social worker to not provide adequate attention to the needs of the client/patient and result in negative consequences.

4. **Critical thinking:** Critical thinking is the ability to analyze information obtained without inclined preferences of observation and communication. Clinical social workers should have the ability to evaluate each case by collecting information through information, interviews, and research. Thinking critically and without prejudice and making informational decisions, identifying the best resources, and formulating the most appropriate intervention plan for clients/patients.

5. **Listen carefully:** Listening carefully is necessary for clinical social workers to understand and identify the needs of customers. Listening carefully, concentrating, asking appropriate questions, using techniques such as paraphrasing and summarizing also helps clinical social workers build trust with their patients.

6. **Personal attention:** Clinical social work can be demanding and emotionally stressful, so it is important to participate in activities that help maintain a balanced life. Personal attention refers to practices that help reduce stress and improve personal well-being, doing these activities helps prevent emotional exhaustion, fatigue and is crucial to a sustainable career. By paying attention to their own person, clinical social workers will be trained to provide the best services to their customers/patients.

7. **Cultural competence:** Effectively working with clients/patients from diverse cultural backgrounds requires clinical social workers to be respectful and respond to cultural and political beliefs. Clinical social workers should have knowledge and respect for cultural histories and as established by the

National Association of Social Workers (2003), examine their own cultural history while seeking necessary knowledge, skills and values that can improve the provision of services to people with a variety of cultural experiences associated with race, ethnicity, education, social class, sexual orientation, religion, age, or disability. By possessing critical attitude and appreciation for diversity and value for individual differences, it helps clinicians to provide patients with what they need.

8. **Patience:** Clinical social workers find several circumstances and individuals in their daily practice. It is important to be clients/patients to work through complex cases and with patients who need long periods of time to progress. This gives clinical social workers power to understand the situation of patients and avoid complicated decisions and frustration that can lead to costly mistakes and poor outcomes for the patient.

9. **Professional commitment:** Being a successful clinical social worker requires a long life of learning. Social workers must have a professional commitment to values and ethics and continue to develop professional competence. This commitment is necessary to achieve the mission of social workers, "to improve human well-being and help meet the basic human needs of all people, with particular attention to the needs of empowering vulnerable, oppressed and living in poverty.

10. **Advocate:** Social workers promote social justice and empower patients and communities through support. The ability to support and skill allows social workers to represent and argue for their clients/patients and connect them with resources and opportunities that are necessary, especially when clients/patients are vulnerable or cannot advocate for themselves.

Theory and Practice Models
Used by Social workers

Introduction:

The author describes the history of social work in England and the United States of America. It also describes theories and mentions the intervention guides that are used by social workers. Social work theories serve as the basis for social work practice by providing an understanding, explanation, and prediction of human behavior.

Chronological History of Social Work:

Social work as a profession originated in the 19th century, mainly in England and the United States. After the end of feudalism, the poor were seen as a threat to the social order, so the state formed and organized a system of help to care for them. In England, the Poor's Law served to classify the poor into different categories: the poor who could work, the disabled, and the raging. This system developed different responses to help these groups of people.

Modern social work in the United States originates during 19th-century mass immigration. Many of the immigrants first arrived in New York and then moved to other cities in the East, where mass conglomeration led to social problems and various diseases. The forerunners of modern social work originated in Elizabeth Blackwell's Medical Dispensary and Jane Adams' Home, while health professionals began working with certain social and health problems (Gehlrt, S; Brown, T.A., 2006; Garcés, C.M., 2002).

As the administration and attitudes of social welfare organizations began to change, so did visiting friends. Just as visiting friends became more systematic and professional, there was general agreement indicating that they needed professional training. In 1981, the Charity movement in New York began publishing and implementing new ideas in this field of practice.

Training programs under the direction of professionals such as Mary Richmond became known around the United States. Mary Richmond pioneered the development of theoretical-methodological proposals for professional intervention and academic training. In 1898, these activities culminated in the establishment of the Summer School for Applied Philanthropy. Immediately afterwards, visiting friends were replaced by professional social workers. At first, new educated and trained visiting friends identified the same as social workers. Early social workers expanded their skills by including another class of social welfare work, expanding the practice of social work cases in child welfare and youth cutting institutions. At the beginning of the twentieth century, voluntary visiting friends from early social welfare organizations developed what is now identified as social case work (Barker, R. L., 1998).

Since the first class of social work was offered by Columbia University in the summer of 1898, social workers have worked developing social welfare organizations to help people in need. Social workers continue to focus on the needs of society and show social problems at national and international level.

The profession of social work is a science because it has as its basis knowledge study and academic research. Social workers can guide their clients/patients, but cannot exercise based on their own opinion and/or style. Social workers study specific clinical theories that are based on research to inform how they are methodologically implemented in clinical practice. Social workers need to obtain both diplomas, Bachelor's and Master's degrees to understand these theories and master the models of theoretical practice.

The approach to social work is in the "person in the environment" (PEA) theory. This considers clients/patients with their psychosocial context and connects them to *micro, mezzo, and macro* levels of social work practice. This guide explores each theory and functions of the practical model within the theory of person in his environment (PEA).

Why is the Use of Theory in Social Work Important?

Understanding clinical theories is an essential part of social work practice (NASW, 2014). This allows social workers to explore certain origins of human behavior with evidence-based interventions. Social workers also make use of these theories and practices to address problems of their clients/patientswith research to support thei rprofessional practice. This is especially important, as social workers need to avoid making personal assumptions or bias that may interfere with the effectiveness of their practice and treatment plan.

Learning about these theories can also help social workers implement effective solutions. If any therapeutic intervention does not work, the social worker can examine the cause and use the one he has learned and treat different interventions.

The Theory of Social Work:

A theory is a group of assumptions, beliefs, or organized ideas about problems in the society where we live. Theory is synonymous with hypotheses, presumptions, speculation, beliefs, ideas and philosophies that is used to help explain or predict situations, actions or consequences. The social work profession intervenes in the place where people live (environment), which requires social workers to have an understanding of the operations and complexities of exercising with different systems. Established theories serve as the basis for explaining human behavior, growth and development, psychological and social functioning, building the social order and ideas of social justice.

Practicing within multiple systems within society makes social work a unique profession. Social work is relatively a new profession. This originated in the 19th century, focusing on the economic and social inequalities that became more prominent after the end of feudalism and the emergence of the industrial revolution. Social workers focused on combating the effects of poverty and promoting social justice. In doing so, social workers needed to understand human behavior, as well as understand the political structures of society and interactions between society and individuals. This need to focus on individuals and the environment in which they live and interact requires the profession to seek in other academic disciplines where the established theories of humans, society and interaction between the two were already established. Therefore, theories within social work are predominantly based on other academic disciplines, such as psychology, sociology, and philosophy (Teater, B., 2010; Turner, F., 2011)

Common Theories in Social Work:

Social workers can incorporate components of different clinical theories into their intervention with clients/patients. Some common interventions of social workers include system theories, social learning, psychosocial development, transpersonal and rational choice. Many of these theories have been developed over the past century and many of them were inspired by Sigmund Freud's theory of psychoanalysis. Some of these theories encompass a broad perspective (such as systems theory), while others focus on specific conflicts (such as social theory). Not all social workers use all theories, but some may use certain elements of each, depending on the circumstances.

Psychodynamic Theory:

This theory was introduced by Sigmund Freud on the turn of the 20th century and was popularized by Carl Jung, Melanie Klein, and Anna Freud. Psychodynamic theory explains that our personality is developed due to various internal forces. Freud wrote that our personality is formed during our early childhood and that our personality consists of three main **parts: id** (impulsive), **ego** (making decisions) and **superego** (consciousness). Psychodynamic theory also prioritizes the process of thinking of a person's unconscious as the root of his behavior.

Function Theory:

Function has its sociological origin from the studies of Cooley, C.H (1902-1909), Mead, H. (1934) and Weber, H. (1947), in the field of psychology and psychiatry. The concept of function can be applied to interaction within the system that also serves as a transition or concept of liaison between individuals and the social system in which it is operating. The concept of function has proven to be conceptual and practically useful and constructive, helping the social science researcher analyze the structure and functions of social systems while explaining the behavior of individuals within these systems (Merton, R., Davidson, K.M, 1990).

Several studies indicate that social workers in hospitals have different expectations and perceptions about their functions and conflict with the definition of social work (Garcés, C., 2002). The role of social workers in the hospital is acquired through socialization and professional certification. Education and preparation for the performance of a professional function is a form of secondary socialization. Primary socialization occurs during childhood and forms fundamental aspects of each person's identity, such as gender, ethnicity, race, and social class functions.

The following concepts of function theory are of importance to social workers, Robbins, S.R. (2008), Merton, R. (1989), Garcés, C., (2002):

1. Certain functions are ordered (by us and for other elements of our social system), in relation to our position within this system.
2. Each function envelops both our own expectations, skills, and other people's expectations.
3. Knowledge of feature expectations implies that there are certain social norms that set the boundaries outside to coincide in conflict-free interactions between positions within the system and between systems.
4. There are values that are emotionally responsible in judging how people should perform their duties, on the part of the person in the position, the role, and others.
5. The concept of function can be used to increase the knowledge base for the use of situation problem assessment.

The discrepancy in the functions of the social worker in the hospital is yet to be resolved. Social workers within the hospital perform roles that are different from those they would like to perform, such as: collaborating with medical staff in patient care; diagnose psychosocial problems, determine patients' eligibility for social services, evaluate and make psychiatric treatment recommendations, help patients recover from the crisis, provide psychotherapy, educate medical staff about social work and psychosocial problems (Garcés, C., 2002).

Rational Choice Theory:

This theory was pioneered by sociologist George, C. Homans in 1950's and states that people make their own decision based on thinking process, especially if those decisions are for their own benefit.

This theory is directly opposed to certain theories that suggest that people make decisions during the unconscious process of thought.

Although rational choice therapy is often found within economics theory, social workers can also apply these principles in their practice. To understand why clients/patients make certain decisions, social workers can examine how these clients/patients believe their decisions could benefit them. Social workers can also develop solutions and suggest resources to help clients/patients achieve their goals.

Social Learning Theory:

This theory was developed by psychologist Albert Bandura. This theory explains how the behavior of certain people affects someone else's behavior. Bandura, A (1977), argues that people learn behaviors by observing and imitating the people around them. Unlike behavioral theories, social learning theory proposes that people actively and mentally process other people's behavior before imitating them (Kurt, S., 2019; Bandura, A., 1977).

Social workers might consider social learning theory when working with children who exhibit violent and aggressive behavior. For example. Children can imitate their parents or other significant adults in their lives. When social workers can identify the origin of a child's behavior, they can effectively create a method of treatment.

Transpersonal Theory:

This theory was developed by Abraham Maslow in 1960, along with Carl Jung and Robert Assagioli. The focus of this theory is holistic philosophy and combines factors such as spirituality, the relationship between the body and the brain and consciousness. Psychologists generally do not consider transpersonal theory as scientific, but many mental health therapists integrate elements of this theory into their practice. They can make use of meditation, mindfulness activities, or hypnotherapy with their clients/patients.

Psychosocial Development Theory:

This theory was influenced by the work of Sigmund Freud. Psychologist Erik Erikson (1987) proposed several stages of development that are related to the identity of the person's ego, personal identity, and social and cultural identity. Erikson's theory argues that humans suffer with specific conflicts through different stages of their lives. These conflicts include:

1. Confidence Vs. mistrust at an early age.
2. Autonomy Vs. Shame and doubt at the early age.
3. Initiative Vs. Guilt.
4. Industrious Vs. Inferiority.
5. Identity Vs. Confusion.
6. Intimacy Vs. Isolation.
7. Generativity Vs. Stagnation.
8. Integrity Vs. Despair.
9. Support Vs. Criticismo.

Crisis Theory:

During the1950s and 1960s, ego psychologists such as Allport, Maslow and Erikson worked on the development of crisis theory. This theory is defined as a group of related concepts that belong to people's reactions when faced with new experiences. These experiences can occur in the form of natural disasters, diseases (Covid-19), significant losses, social, economic changes and life cycles. This theory suggests that when people face situations such as trauma, they have a tendency to follow predictable response patterns (Ell, K., 1995; Golan, A. L., 1978).). Crisis theory developed because of the concern of people who temporarily feel feelings of distress or not being able to adapt to life's problems and emotional stress events (Covid-19).

Crisis intervention is important for social workers who daily find many of their clients/patients in hospitals (emergency rooms, ICU, mental health clinics), in situations of emotional trauma, unease and anxiety. Providing appropriate interventions to people in emotional crises is part of the daily practice of social workers and crisis intervention is in the legitimate interest of social workers.

The social work practice encompasses a process that determines professional intervention, about what needs to be done, how to do it and in what or rden, to ensure that people can overcome the crisis that is affecting them.

Social worker intervention in crisis situations is important for the following reasons:

1. Identifies and controls crisis situations.
2. Provides crisis interventions.
3. Promotes interventions to relieve specific symptoms and reduce emotional stress.
4. Assess the environmental reaction and connect the victim, family, and caregivers (doctors, nurses), with community service resources.
5. Identifies psychosocial interventions.
6. Evaluates and monitors psychosocial aspects of pain/penalty.
7. Assess the effectiveness of crisis intervention.

Scientific Theory:

The main objective of this theory is to examine and criticize political structures and functioning and their effects on individuals, families, and communities (Payne, M., 2005). Such policies and understanding of social structures and policies will assist social workers in working to address inequalities and disadvantages and promote social justice.

Conflict theory is a form of scientific theory, which is based on the work of Karl Marx and Max Weber, whose focus on inequalities within society, such as wealth, power, social class, and how such inequalities impact the experiences of a person's life. And possibilities to create conflict between and with social groups (Hier, S. P., 2005). Several theories have been applied to the practice of social work with the intention of recognizing the inequalities and disadvantages that clients can and experience within the current political and social structures promote a course of action and interventions that may challenge such inequalities.

Systems Theory:

This theory assumes that human behavior is the result of an extensive system consisting of several elements, including the relationship between these elements, as well as external factors such as their environment. These factors may include the family of individuals, friends, school, place of employment, or community. Sociologists have identified different types of systems, including *microsystems, meso systems, exosystems and macrosystems.* Systems theory is based on the belief that individuals do not operate isolated, on the contrary, they grow and develop in interaction with their physical and social environment. Systems theory is derived from general systems theory, which explores the parts of a system that interconnects and interacts with the purpose of making a complete whole (Teater, B., 2010). Within social work, systems can constitute individuals, couples, families, communities, organizations, society, and the world. Systems theory suggests that each system should be seen as a consisting of several elements that make the system fully functioning and that each system should consider the biopsicosocial aspects of the client by observing the physical and psychological functioning, social relationships and structures of the community or society that impact the client.

Micro, Vs. Mezzo, Vs. Social Work Guide Work (2020):

Social workers perform their roles and responsibilities within three interrelated levels in their practice: micro, mezzo, and macro. These practice systems use different methodologies to provide services to diverse populations, but all operate within the Person-Environment Theory (PEA). Based on the importance of the environmental factors of human behavior, the PAE provides the structure of social work practice. This theoretic premise connects the three systems, and helps social workers understand the complex set of social factors that affect their clients/patients.

Because the social work field offers versatile options and specializations, social workers often integrate different levels of practice, while working with multiple systems to effectively assist their clients/patients. While educational qualifications, undergraduate requirements, and the different types of careers associated with each practice system could overlap, each level represents a distinctive discipline. This guide can help future social workers understand the three practice systems, including how these can impact educational options and career prospects.

Micro Social Work:

Typically, micro social work describes the individualized approach that is used by clinical social workers providing direct services, interventions and support to individuals, families, and groups. These social workers provide one-on-one psychotherapy and assessments to small groups in a variety of therapeutic locations, including hospitals, mental health centers, schools, nursing homes, prisons. The micro level is commonly associated with traditional clinical social work, which addresses the social needs of the most vulnerable groups in society, including children, older adults, victims of domestic violence and those with emotional problems. Social workers evaluate systems where clients/patients live affects their behavior. For example, living in a poverty system can have a significant impact on how a person makes decisions. Social workers can create strategies based on these systems to provides more concise treatment model for their clients/patients.

Mezzo Social Work Model:

Although most social workers offer direct individual services, their primary focus is on solving problems in favor of customer groups, or "customer system." These social workers identify factors that affect the well-being of many clients/patients within organizations such as schools or social services agencies, or within small communities, such as at-risk youth in neighborhoods within the city.

"Mezzo" social workers collaborate with other client and agency systems, implementing programs and advocating for services and resources. "M*icro" social* workers often participate in "mezzo"levels of social work to help their clients achieve their goals. For example, school counselors can develop a workshop program to prevent illicit drug abuse to benefit students with these problems.

Macro Social Work:

The*"macro"* social work model focuses on the challenge of alleviating social problems and improving people's quality of life at the local, national, and international levels. For many people who are not familiar with this field of intervention, the level of "macro" social work could not be recognized as social work. Social workers at the "macro" level can contribute to the development of laws or petitions at the local, state level, as well as in government funds to help communities. Activities and activities can also be organized at national and international level.

Macro social workers investigate the origin, persistence, and impact of social problems on the population, such as homelessness or suicide in young people; create and implement initiatives for social services and address social problems, including opium crises, or diabetes on children; advocate for promoting policy changes and legislation to benefit vulnerable populations, such as expanding access to health benefits for low-income people.

Common Models in the Social Work Policy (NASW, 2014):

While social workers can integrate various clinical theories into their practice, they can also implement specific therapeutic models. The above theories may explain the causes of a person's problems, therefore, the models of policy allow social workers to apply specific interventions for the treatment of certain problems. So some social workers specialize in a single aspect of micro-macro scale, many social workers interact with all three levels. In this way, social workers must understand the full spectrum and how these models of intervention interact.

The following section describes some of the most common models of social work practice, including cognitive therapy, behavior*therapy, crisis intervention, narrative therapy, problem-solving model, solution therapy approach, and task focus therapy.* Some of these methods share characteristics among themselves, but each has a specific purpose for each client/patient and their circumstances.

Cognitive Behavior Therapy:

This therapy (CBT) identifies thought patterns and tries to rewrite these patterns. People are often convinced that their frequent and distorted thoughts are true. Cognitive behavior therapy forces people to confront these distortions. For example, someone may be afraid in social situations, imagining themselves in humiliating situations for them. The TCC forces the person to examine these assumptions and consider new scenarios and landscapes. People suffering from anxiety and depression discover that this therapy helps them, and many social workers incorporate it into their therapeutic practice.

Crisis Intervention Model:

The model of crisis intervention is more than it seems: in times of acute tension or psychosocial stress, social workers intervene before the crisis causes harm to the person in crisis. Psychologists Albert Roberts and Allen Ottens proposed several steps to take in crisis intervention. These include conducting a safety assessment, establishing psychological contact, identifying major problems, helping the client/patient explore their feelings/emotions, seeking new defense mechanisms, creating a treatment and follow-up plan. Social workers can use the crisis intervention model with clients/patients who have suffered trauma and post-trauma disorders, suicidal thoughts, among others. The crisis intervention model works on a voluntary basis, which means that clients/patients must cooperate during this process.

Narrative Therapy Model:

This therapy is based on the theory that the person changes their personal experiences into stories. Creating narratives of their own lives (Madigan, S., 2011). This kind of therapy is based on four main principles: "Objective truth," which does not exist, reality is a social construct, language can influence the way we see reality and narratives help us organize our personal realities. Narrative therapy encourages clients/patients to distance the therself from their personal experiences by adopting the role of a narrator and rewriting the libretto. This can help them change dangerous and destructive thoughts, especially those that caused them emotional trauma.

Troubleshooting Therapy Model:

Hellen Harris Perlman proposed this model in the 1950s, especially for the field of social work. During that time, many theories of social work and therapies relied on psychotherapy. They instead argued that social workers could be more efficient in helping clients/patients by focusing on one problem at a time.

Focusing on minor problems allows clients/patients to develop and follow action plans to address these problems in a manageable manner. This model, also called "partialization," can make therapy more manageable for both social workers and clients/patients. Many social workers use Perlman's proposal.

Solution-Centered Therapy:

This therapy focuses on short, concentration therapy in the person's present and in future situations (Watson, J., 2006). Solution-focused therapy involves the separation of therapies influenced by psychodynamic theory, whose focus is on a person's past and childhood.

Solution-focused therapy proposes immediate solutions that are manageable, allowing the customer/patient to do better in the face of problems. Social workers who use this type of therapy can challenge the client/patient to imagine their future life smoothly, or they can also help them better recognize the defense mechanisms they had previously used. Likewise, social workers in mental health can implement this theory in adolescents with behavioral problems, with people with emotional problems, as well as with conflicting families.

Focused Policy Tasks Model:

This technique shares many principles with the problem solving and approach model, as this technique tries to follow a quick approach. Focused Policy Tasks usually last a period of 8-12 sessions and the client/patient focuses on achieving measurable goals. The client/patient and social worker develop an action plan with specific tasks, and then clients/patients continue to do these tasks alone. Social workers can integrate this type of therapy into different places. They can work with students who have disruptive behaviors, with clients/patients who are about to be discharged from the hospital, with older adults in nursing homes.

Biographical References

Abraido-Lanza, Armbrister, A.N. (2006). Towards a theory driven model of acculturation. PubMed.

Altena, E., Baglioni, C., Espie, CA., Ellis, J., Gavriloff, D., Holzinger, B. (2020). Dealing with sleep problems during home confinement due to theCovid-19 outbreak: Practical recommendations from a task force of the European CBT-I Academy. Sleep res.

Arredondo, P. (1999). Multicultural counseling competencies as tools to address oppression and racism. Journal Counseling and Development.

Asamoah, Y. (1996). Innovations in delivering culturally sensitive social work services. New York: Haworth Press.

Bandura, (1977). Social Learning Theory. Englewood Cliffs, NJ: Prentice.

Barker, R. L., 1998). Milestones in the Development of Social Work and Social Welfare. Washington, DC: NASW.

Barker, R.L. (2003). The Social Work Dictionary 5th ed. Washington, DC: NASW.

Bernal, G., Saez-Santiago. S. (2006). Culturally Centered Psychosocial Interventions. Journal of Community Psychology.

Boyer, P. (2001). Cultural Assimilation. International Encyclopedia of the Social Sciences and Behavioral Sciences.

Comas-Diaz, L. (2010). Multicultural Approaches to Psychotherapy (2011). Interventions with Culturally Diverse Population. Oxford.

Cooley, Ch. H. (1902). Human Nature and the Social Order. New York: Charles Scriber's Sons.

Council on Social Work Education (CSWE). (2015). Educational Policy and Accreditation Standards. Retrieved from; http://www.cswe.org/getatachement/Accreditation/Accreditation Process/2015-EPAS-Web-Final.pdf.aspx

Davidson, K. (1990). Role Blurring and the Hospital Social Worker's Search for Domain. Health and Social Work., 15, pp.228-234.

Department of Health (2003). Delivering Race inequality: A Framework for Action. London: Department of Health.

Diagnostic and Statistical Manual of Mental Disorders (DSM-V 2013). American Psychiatric Association. Fifth Edition.

Elke Van Hoof (2020). Coronavirus and Quarantine: Confinement is the Greatest Psychological Experiment in History.

Erik Erikson (1987). The Life Cycle. Completed: A Review, New York: W. W. Norton. pp. 32-33.

Escobar, F., Quijano, m., Calvo, J. (2017). Evaluation of Insomnia as a Risk Factor for Suicide. Rev Fac Hundred Med. 74 (1): 37-45.

Garcés C.M. (2002). Doctoral dissertation. The Social Worker in the Emergency Room. Yeshiva University. New York.

Garcés, C. (2018). The Intervention of the Social Worker in the Hospital Center-Challenges for the Profession. Revised Edition. Palibrio.

Gehler, S., Brown, A. (2006). Chapter Two; The Conceptual Underpinning of Social Work. New Jersey: Wiley.

German, P., Seelig, A.D., Jacobson, I.G., Boyko, E.J., Hooper, T.I., Gackstetter, G.D. (2013). Redeployment Sleep Duration and Insomnia Symptoms as Risk factors for New Onset Mental Health Disorders Fallowing Military Deployment. Sleep. 36 (7): 1009-1018.

Golan, A. (1978). Crisis Intervention. New York: Free Press.

Hier, S. P. (2005). Contemporary Sociological Thought: Themes and Theories. Toronto, Canadian Scholar's Press.

Hwan, Wei-Chin (2006). The Psychotherapy adaptation and Modification Framework: application to Asian Americans.

Imaginary, A. (2000). Meaning of Culture.

International Federation of Social Workers (2020). Calls for Mental health for All.

Jani, Jayshee, S., Ortiz, A., & Aranda, M. (2008). Latino Outcomes on Social Work Practice.

Journal of clinical Psychology (2010): In Session, Vol. 66(8), 821-829

Kaiser Family Foundation (2020). The implications of Covid 19 for Mental Health and Substance Use. https:www.kff.org/ healthreform/issue-brief/the-implications-of-covid19-for-mental-healthand-substance-use/?utm-campain+KFF.extraidojunio20/2020

Kira, P. Kira. J (2004). What do Patients Receiving Palliative Care for Cancer and Their Families Want to be Told? An Australian and Canadian Qualitative Study. B. M. J: 328-1343

Kirwan, M., Pickett, S.M., Jarret, N.L. (2017). Emotion regulation as a moderator between anxiety symptoms and insomnia symptom severity. Psychiatry Res. 1; 254: 40-47.

Kumpfer, K. L., Alvarado, R., Smith, P., Bellamy, N. (2002). Cultural Sensitivity and adaptation. PubMed.

Kurt, S. (2019). Social Learning Theory: Albert Bandura, "In Educational Technology." Retrieved from: https://educationaltechnology.net/social-learning-theory-albert-bandura/

Lai J, Ma S, Wang Y, and colleagues (2020). Factors associated with Mental Health Outcome Among Health Care Workers Exposed to Coronavirus Disease. JAMA New Open. 3(3): e203976

Liu, W.M., & Ali, S. R. (2005). Addressing social class and classism in vocational theory and practice: Extending the emancipatory communitarian approach. Counseling Psychologist, 33, 189-196., Mental Health Atlas. (2017).

Lopez, S.R., Grover, K.P., Holland., Johnson, M.J., Kain, C.D., Kanel, K., (1989). Development of culturally sensitive psychotherapists. Professional Psychology: Research and Practice. Pp. 169-135. Washington, DC: American Psychosocial Association.

Madigan, S. (2011). Narrative Therapy. American Psychological Association.

McGuire, T. G., & Miranda, J. (2008). New evidence regarding racial and ethnic disparities in mental health: Policy implications. Health Affairs, 27(2), 393-403.

Mead, G. H. (1934). Self and Society. Chicago: University Press of Chicago Press.

Merton, R. (1957). Social Theory and Social Structure. New York: free Press.

Micro vs. Mezzo, vs. Macro Social Work (2020). Retrieved from: https:/www.socialworkguide.org/resources/micro-vs.mezzo-vs-macro-social-work/

My Lee 92003). Focused Task Model. Families in Society.

National Association of Social Workers (2014). Common Models in Social Work Practice. NASW. Washington DC: Author.

Norries, F., & Joy, M. (2005). Mental health for minority individuals and communities in the aftermath of disasters and mass violence. CNS Spectrums, 10, 132-140.

Pearson, Katherine (2020) The First data on Covid-19 and Teens' Mental health is Here- And is Not Good. Re-copied on June 26 (2020). https://www.huffpost.com/entry-the-first-data- on-covid-19-and-teens-mental-health-is-and-its-not-good

Poole, D. L., & Salgado de Snyder, V. N. (2002). Pathways to health and mental health care: Guidelines for culturally competent practice. In A. R. Roberts & G. J. Greene (Eds). Social workers' desk reference (pp. 51-56). New York: Oxford University Press.

Psychology and Spanish Elective Opportunity (PASEO) (2010).

Robbins, S.P. (2008). Organizational Theory. Structure, design, and Implications. San Diego State University. Prentice Hall. Englewood Cliffs, New Jersey

Rogers, L-Sirin, P. Rice, S. R., Sirin. (2014). Acculturation and cultural mismatch and their Influences on immigrant children and Adolescents' Wellbeing.

Schwartzbaum, S.E. (2004). Low-income Latinos and dropout: Strategies to prevent dropout. Journal of Multicultural Counseling and Development, 32, 296-306.

Smedley, B.D.S., Stith, A.Y., Nelson, E.R. (2003). Unequal Treatment. Confronting Racial and Ethnic Disparities in Health Care. Washington, DC: National Academic Press.

Social Work. Chicago, IL: Lyceum Books; Google Scholar.

Sue, D. W. Arredondo, P. & McDavis, R. (1992). Multicultural competency and standards: A call to the profession. Journal of Multicultural Counseling and Development, 20.64-88.

Sue, D. W., & Sue, D. (1990). Counseling the culturally different: Theory and Practice (2nd. ed). New York: John Wiley and Sons.

Sue, D. W., Rasheed, J.M. (2015). Multicultural Social Work Practice: A competency-based approach to diversity and social justice (2nded.). Hoboken, N.J: John Wiley & Sons, INC.

Taylor, B.A., Beatriz-Gambourg, M., Rivera, M., & Laureano. D. (2006). Constructing cultural competence perspectives of family therapists working with Latino Families. American Journal of Family Therapy, 34, 429-445.

Teater, B. (2010). An Introduction to Applying Social Work Theories and Methods. Maidenhead, Open University Press.

The Harris Poll (2020). National 4-H Council

The President's Initiative on Race. Pathways to one America in the 21st Century. Washington, DC: US Government Printing Office.

Tom, David (1995). Psychiatry. Fifth Edition. Williams & Wilkins.

Torres, L. & Rollock, D. (2004). Acculturative distress among Hispanics: The role of acculturation, coping, and intercultural competence. Journal of Multicultural Counseling and Development, 32, 155-167.

Turner, F. (2011). Theory and Social Work Treatment, in: F. Turner (Ed.). Social Work Treatment: Interlocking Theoretical Approaches. Oxford University Press, pp-3-14.

University of Buffalo (2021). Essential Skills and Traits for Social Workers.

Virruel-Fuentes, E. A., Miranda, P. Y., & Abdulrain, S. (2012). More than culture: Structural racism, intersectionality. Theory, and immigrant health. Social Science & Medicine, 75(12), 2099-2106.

Watson, C. Jeanne (2006). Educational Publishing Foundation. 43(1) 13.

Weber, M.ax. (1947). The Theory of Social and Economic Organizations, ed., Talcott Parsons, Trans. AM. Henderson, and Talcott Parsons. New York Press.

Wilkinson-Lee, A., Russell, S. T., & Lee, F.C. H. (2006). Practitioners' perspectives on cultural sensitivity in Latino/a teen pregnancy prevention. Family Relations. 55(3),376-389.

Williams, C.C. (2006). The epistemology of cultural competence. Families in Society, 87(2),209-220.

World culture report (2000). Cultural Diversity, Conflict and Pluralism. Corporate author: UNESCO. Director-General, 1999-2009 (Matsura, K.)

World Health Organization (2020). Covid-19. Strategy Update. https://www.who.int/docs/default-source/coronavirus/covid-strategyupdate-14april2020.pdf?extraido June21/2020

World Health Organization-WHO (2014). Mental Health: A State of Wellbeing. Author.

Zayas, L.H. Torres, L.R., Malcolm, J., & Desrasim (1996). Clinicians' definitions of ethnically therapy.

Zea, M.C.., Asner-Self, K.K., Burmese, D., & Buki, L., P. (2003). The abbreviated multidimensional acculturation scale: Empirical validation with two Latino/Latina samples. Cultural Diversity and ethnic Minority Psychology: 9, 107-126.

Zhang, C., yang, L., Liu, S., Wang, Y., Cai, Z. (2020). Survey of Insomnia and Related Social Psychological Factors Among Medical Staff Involved in the 2019 Novel Coronavirus Disease Outbreak. 14-11.